LABORATORY MANUAL

Selected Experiments of
Pharmaceutical Analysis

W0080585

Second Edition

As per the latest B Pharm I M Pharm syllabi
prescribed by Pharmacy Council of India

LABORATORY MANUAL
Selected Experiments of
Pharmaceutical
Analysis

Second Edition

As per the latest B Pharm | M Pharm syllabi
prescribed by Pharmacy Council of India

Anees Ahmad Siddiqui M Pharm PhD
Professor
BM College of Pharmacy
Gurugram, Haryana
Ex Professor and Head
Department of Pharmaceutical Chemistry
School of Pharmaceutical Education and Research
Jamia Hamdard
New Delhi

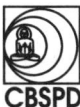

CBSPD

CBS Publishers & Distributors Pvt Ltd

New Delhi • Bengaluru • Chennai • Kochi • Kolkata • Lucknow • Mumbai
Hyderabad • Jharkhand • Nagpur • Patna • Pune • Uttarakhand

LABORATORY MANUAL
Selected Experiments of
Pharmaceutical Analysis
Second Edition

ISBN: 978-93-89261-76-9

Copyright © Author and Publisher

Second Edition: 2020
Reprint: 2024
First Edition: 2010

Published by Satish Kumar Jain and produced by Varun Jain for
CBS Publishers & Distributors Pvt Ltd
4819/XI Prahlad Street, 24 Ansari Road, Daryaganj, New Delhi 110 002, India.
Ph: 011-23289259, 23266838   Website: www.cbspd.com
                                   e-mail: delhi@cbspd.com

Corporate Office: 204 FIE, Industrial Area, Patparganj, Delhi-110092
Ph: 011-4934 4934   Fax: 011-4934 4935   e-mail: publishing@cbspd.com; publicity@cbspd.com

Branches

- **Bengaluru:** Seema House 2975, 17th Cross, K.R. Road, Banasankari 2nd Stage, Bengaluru 560 070, Karnataka, India
  Ph: +91-80-26771678/79   Fax: +91-80-26771680   e-mail: bangalore@cbspd.com
- **Chennai:** 7, Subbaraya Street, Shenoy Nagar, Chennai 600 030, Tamil Nadu
  Ph: +91-44-26680620, 26681266   Fax: +91-44-42032115   e-mail: chennai@cbspd.com
- **Kochi:** 42/1325, 1326, Power House Road, Opp KSEB Power House, Ernakulam 682 018, Kochi, Kerala, India
  Ph: +91-484-4059061-65   Fax: +91-484-4059065   e-mail: kochi@cbspd.com
- **Kolkata:** 147, Hind Ceramics Compound, 1st Floor, Nilgunj Road, Belghoria, Kolkata 700 056, West Bengal, India
  Ph: +91-033-25633055, 033-25633056   e-mail: kolkata@cbspd.com
- **Lucknow:** Basement, Khushnuma Complex, 7-Meerabai Marg (behind Jawahar Bhawan), Lucknow 226 001, UP, India
  Ph: +91-522-400043, 9919002738   e-mail: tiwari.lucknow@cbspd.com
- **Mumbai:** PWD Shed, Gala no. 25/26, Ramchandra Bhatt Marg, Next to JJ Hospital Gate no. 2
  Opp. Union Bank of India, Noorbaug, Mumbai-400009, Maharashtra, India
  Ph: 022-60061880/89   e-mail: mumbai@cbspd.com

Representatives

• **Hyderabad**	0-9885175004	• **Jharkhand**	0-9811541605	• **Nagpur**	0-8692091830
• **Patna**	0-9334159340	• **Pune**	0-9664372571	• **Uttarakhand**	0-9716462459

Printed at: Mudrak, Noida, UP (India)

Preface to the Second Edition

Pharmaceutical analytical chemistry is a subject of experimental science. Thus, it is important that students of pharmaceutical chemistry do experiments in the laboratory to understand the theories they study in lecture and in their textbook and do the critical evaluation of experimental data. Conclusively, experimentation allows students to develop better selective, sensitive and more accurate methods for qualitative and quantitative analysis of pharmaceutical substances.

The analytical chemistry experiments in this laboratory manual entitled *Selected Experiments of Pharmaceutical Analysis* are designed to follow the pharmacy curriculum of undergraduate and postgraduate courses. However, instructors sometimes vary the order of material covered in lecture and, thus, certain experiments may come before the concepts illustrated are covered in lecture or after the material has been covered. Some instructors strongly feel that the lecture should lead the laboratory while other instructors just as strongly believe that the laboratory experiments should lead the lecture, and still a third group feel that they should be done concurrently. While there is no "best" way, it is important that you carefully prepare for each experiment by reading the related text material before coming to the laboratory. In this way, you can maximize the laboratory experience, and can, thus, develop the analytical skill.

Laboratory experiments are categorized according to type of titration or techniques. Each technique is introduced before experiments. In most of the laboratory experiments, molar solutions are used as followed in recent edition of *Indian Pharmacopoeia*. *Viva voce* type of questions are included in each experiment to prepare the students for practical examination.

In the present edition, some experiments have been added. Two chapters "Differential Scanning Colorimetry" and "High Performance Thin Layer Chromatography" have also been added along with relevant experiments.

The typographic mistakes prevailing in previous edition have been rectified. I acknowledge Dr Sharmistha Mohapatra and Dr Jamshed Haneef and other colleagues for their special assistance in bringing out this second edition.

I am thankful to Dr Rajiv Tonk and Ravinesh Mishra for their valuable suggestions. I am thankful to Mr SK Jain CMD, CBS Publishers & Distributors Pvt Ltd, New Delhi, for his cooperation in bringing out this second edition.

Anees Ahmad Siddiqui

Preface to the First Edition

Pharmaceutical chemistry is an experimental science. Thus, it is important that students of pharmaceutical chemistry do experiments in the laboratory to more fully understand that the theories they study in lecture and in their textbook, developed from the critical evaluation of experimental data. The laboratory can also aid the student in the study of the science by clearly illustrating the principles and concepts involved. Finally, laboratory experimentation allows students the opportunity to develop techniques and other manipulative skills that students of science must master.

The experiments in this laboratory manual entitled *Selected Experiments of Pharmaceutical Analysis* is designed to follow the pharmacy curriculum. However, instructors will sometimes vary the order of material covered in lecture and thus certain experiments may come before the concepts illustrated are covered in lecture or after the material has been covered. Some instructors strongly feel that the lecture should lead the laboratory while other instructors just as strongly believe that the laboratory experiments should lead the lecture, and still a third group feel that they should be done concurrently. While there is no "best" way, it is important that you carefully prepare for each experiment by reading the related text material before coming to the laboratory. In this way you can maximize the laboratory experience.

Laboratory experiments are categorized according to type of titration or techniques. Each technique is introduced before experiments. In most of the Laboratory experiments, molar solutions are used as followed in recent edition of *Indian Pharmacopoeia*. Questions are presented throughout each experiment. It is important that you try to answer each question, as it will help you understand the experiment as you do it. Appendices are also included in last for reference at a glance.

I acknowledge Mr Vijay Kumar, Director, JASVIC Laboratories, Roorki (UK) for his special assistance in designing the instrumental experiments.

I am thankful to Mr Rajiv Tonk and Ravinesh Mishra for their valuable suggestion.

I am also thankful to Mr SK Jain and Mr Vinod K Jain for their cooperation to bring out this manual.

Anees Ahmad Siddiqui

Contents

Introduction

Reagents

Reagents are supplied in the manufacturer's bottles. Note the analysis reported (or analytical report) on the label on reagent bottle. Record the manufacturer and grade of the reagent (e.g. lab grade or analytical grade) used in your lab notebook. This information is always required in writing a technical paper and you should get in the habit of recording it.

The purity of the reagents used is a determining factor in getting perfect results in analytical determination. Consequently, every effort must be made to keep stock bottles free from contamination. Under no circumstances should unused material be returned to a stock bottle in a general laboratory. A large stainless steel scoopula with a handle or a porcelain spatula may be used to break up caked solids.

In general, solids are best poured from bottles. Rotating the bottle back and forth helps to control the rate of flow. Droppers and pipettes should never be dipped into stock bottles. Droppers from dropper bottles should not come in contact with any surface outside of the dropper bottle itself.

Primary standards

Substances prepared for use as primary standards are so labelled for their appropriate use. These materials are expensive and must not be used for routine procedures.

Drying at elevated temperatures

Drying ovens for these analytical exercises are thermostated and are usually operated at 120–125°C. As the name implies, they are used for drying at an elevated temperature. The efficiency of the drying process also depends upon the pressure of water vapor in the immediate atmosphere. Consequently, a very wet object introduced into an oven may actually cause another object in the same oven to pick up water. Consequently, one should not place wet glassware in an oven being used to dry analytical samples or standards. Before using the ovens, note the temperature at which they are operating. Do not change the setting on an oven without consulting the instructor.

Cleaning glassware

The cleaning process should be as simple as possible. Rinsing with tap water and several small portions of distilled water may be adequate. For more dirty glassware, scrubbing with detergent and water should precede the rinsing. Always use soft brushes with wooden or soft plastic handle to avoid abrasion. From a chemical point of view, soap, detergents, etc. are dirt. Rinse very thoroughly with tap water and then at least three times with small volumes of distilled water. In a few cases, special chemicals may be needed to dissolve solids or oils. The inside of a container which may come in contact with chemicals is not dried with a towel since this introduces lint. In many cases, it is not necessary to dry glassware. Simply rinse with the solution to be used unless this would invalidate measurements. Beware of drying glassware with compressed air. This may introduce oil vapor from the pump. Always wash glassware immediately after use. If a thorough cleaning is not immediately possible, always allow the glassware to soak. If not cleaned immediately, some residues may be impossible to remove.

Chromic acid cleaning solutions

A solution of potassium dichromate dissolved in concentrated sulfuric acid was traditionally used for difficult cleaning tasks. The use of this solution should be avoided as chromium compounds are Class I carcinogens.

Glassware which resists cleaning with lab soap and water may be cleaned with other special cleaning solutions. For trace metal analysis, it is common practice to soak glassware in 50% nitric acid solution. When placing glassware into such a bath, it is important not to be splashed by the bath. When removing glassware, long, chemically resistant gloves must be worn. Do not use tongs for this job as they are dissolved by the bath. Glassware must be removed and rinsed in a manner that does not leave hazardous acid residues in the work area which other people may be exposed to.

Removal of grease

Grease is best removed by boiling the glass in a weak solution of sodium carbonate. Acetone or other organic solvent can also be used.

Cleaning volumetric glassware

Volumetric glassware must be clean so that water drains from the surface without leaving droplets. It is not possible if there is even a bit of oil on the surface. Once "clean" glassware becomes dry, it will usually not drain properly when water is again added. Volumetric glassware is cleaned just before use or cleaned and stored full of distilled water or other solvent.

Working surfaces

Use paper towels to wipe up all spilled materials. Repeatedly wash the surface with a wet towel to remove water soluble materials including acids and bases. The working surface should be kept clean and dry. Spilled material is then quite evident and contamination can be kept at a minimum. If working materials are arranged in an organized manner, there are fewer opportunities for confusion and there is a higher probability that a determination will be carried through to completion without error.

Quantitative transfer

Quantitative transfer is the complete transfer of a sample without loss of any kind. The techniques used are a matter of common sense—do not spill, splash, or abandon. Dry solids are poured or transferred with a spatula. If the surface tension of a liquid is high it should be transferred by pouring down a stirring rod. This prevents the liquid from running down the outside of the original container and also prevents splashing as the liquid enters the second container. Last traces are transferred by washing the original container and transfer equipment such as spatula, stirring rod and funnel with a miscible liquid. This can be done by a batch method using repeated small volumes of the wash liquid or by a continuous flow method using a stream of wash liquid from a wash bottle. A rubber policeman is used to facilitate the process and minimize the amount of wash solution necessary. Transfer of material from a weighing bottle to a flask should always be done by pouring and not with a spatula.

Weighing of samples

The preferred method is known as weighing by difference, is to weigh the weighing bottle containing the dry sample, transfer the sample to the flask in which it is to be used, and reweigh the weighing bottle. This last weight becomes the first weight for a second sample if multiple samples are being prepared. This method assumes that the receiver flask has a large enough opening that there is minimal risk for spillage. The receiver flask need not be dry, so considerable time can be saved through not needing to dry glassware. When transferring from a weighing bottle to a volumetric flask, a powder funnel should be used to facilitate transfer. For solids, a powder funnel with a wide and short stem is more appropriate as it does not clog easily.

Samples can be added to a clean dry container, often a weighing boat, which has been previously weighed or tared on the balance. Extreme care must be taken when samples are transferred from this container to insure that no material is lost. Normally, the solvent should be used to wash any residue from the boat into the container at the end of the transfer. Caution must be exercised with the common plastic boats as they can accumulate static electricity which either attracts or repels the particles of sample. This method is not recommended for the most precise quantitative work.

The best way to manipulate the weighing bottle is to use a band of dry paper pulled firmly around the bottle. Do not use your fingers directly on the weighing bottle as the moisture from your fingers will affect the weight. If the weighing bottle stands for several hours in the desiccator before taking the next sample, its weight should be rechecked.

Rules for use of analytical balances

Operate all balances gently, especially after reading the instructions. You should know the names and functions of all the controls. Weighing on the analytical balances should never be done on weighing paper (or filter paper, paper towels, etc.). If sufficient precision is demanded to require the analytical balance, it also requires the use of procedures which do not involve such high risk of loss during transfer. The second problem with use of paper is that it leads to dirty, and subsequently, damaged balances. Acceptable weighing containers are weighing bottles, plastic weighing boats, and glassware with sides to contain the material.

No reagent shall be added to or subtracted from a container while in the analytical balance. Remove the container to the bench top, make the addition and return to the balance.

Heating and concentrating solutions

Aqueous solutions may be heated either on a Bunsen burner with wire gauze or on the hot plates. The burner is often a quicker method for rapid heating while the hot plate will provide a constant level of heat for a long time. Solutions other than water or dilute aqueous salts should be heated in the hoods. A watch glass should always be used during the heating of solutions both to prevent entry of extraneous material from your neighbors sample, the paint on the ceiling, etc., and to prevent loss of sample due to splattering. Ordinary watch glasses restrict the loss of vapor and are used to maintain the value of the solution. When evaporation is desirable the watch glass may be supported with three glass hooks or ribbed watch glasses may be used. These allow escape of vapors. In either case, some sample will collect on the watch glass and must be rinsed back into the container with a small volume of the solvent whenever the watch glass is removed. Boiling is generally to be avoided with samples due to the high risk of mechanical loss. When boiling is desired, boiling chips (glass beads or chips, marble chips, silicon carbide) should be used whenever possible.

Handling Stock Solutions

A uniformly mixed solution may develop a concentration gradient on standing even in a closed bottle. Evaporation occurs from the surface of the liquid. Condensation takes place on the wall of the container above the surface and the condensate flows down the wall into the solution again. Shake or mix stock solutions before use.

Control Charts

Control chart is used to evaluate the consistency of the procedures you are using. This procedure is used in most routine labs. Place the charts in the lab and enter your data before you leave the lab at the end of each day.

VOLUMETRIC GLASSWARE

Flasks, Burets and Pipets

The specifications used by most of the manufacturers of volumetric glassware meet the specified standard. Measurements of volumes larger than 10 ml. can easily be made with an accuracy of 1 or 2 parts per thousand. Smaller volumes, which are so much a part of present day chemistry, may present special problems.

Since the volume of a container depends upon the temperature, volumetric equipment is calibrated for a specified temperature—usually 20°C. The coefficient of expansion of glass is so small that calibrations for 20°C are valid over the usual range of laboratory temperatures. Even at 30°C the error is less than 0.3 ppt. Tolerances for various pieces of equipment have been recommended. For example, the tolerance for a 50 ml. flask or a 50 ml. transfer pipet is 0.05 ml. Properly used volume is 50.00 ± 0.05 ml. This is a maximum error of 1 ppt. The tolerance for a 10 ml transfer pipet is 0.02 ml, 2 ppt. Note that for the smaller volume the tolerance is proportionally larger although smaller in absolute magnitude.

Graduated cylinders

Graduate cylinders should not be used for any quantitative measurement which is part of an analytical determination. They are useful for preparing stock solutions, HPLC mobile phases, and other places where the accuracy of the measurement does not have a direct contribution to the quantitative calculation. Graduated cylinders are very crude pieces of volumetric equipment. Non-uniformity of glass at the base of the cylinder makes the measurement of small volumes of liquid in the bottom of the cylinder particularly unreliable.

Graduated measuring pipets

Measuring pipets look like a buret without a stopcock. They are frequently convenient to use but should in no sense be considered as precision equipment—largely due to the difficulty in controlling the level of the liquid. In normal use they are no better than graduate cylinders and should not be used quantitatively unless errors greater than 10% relative are expected in the results.

Volumetric transfer pipets

A transfer pipet has a single calibration line on tubing of small diameter and is capable of high precision. It is, however, frequently used incorrectly and becomes a serious source of error. For this reason an operator should run enough calibration checks to attain self confidence in their technique as well as confidence in the equipment.

All transfer pipets in the lab should be marked. The proper use of these pipets is as follows:

(i) Fill the pipet above the calibration line using a bulb. Mouth pipeting is not allowed and will result in expulsion from the lab.

(ii) Tip the pipet to an angle to prevent leakage

(iii) Wipe excess liquid from the outer surface of the pipet with a clean towel or wipe.

(iv) Drain the pipet until the liquid level reaches the calibration line.

(v) Touch the tip of the pipet to a glass surface to remove the attached drop which is probably present.

(vi) Tilt the pipet to carry it to the receiving vessel. This will prevent loss of sample.

(vii) Drain the contents into the receiving vessel. Do not force the liquid out. Let it take its time.

(viii) After the pipet has stopped draining for 10–20 seconds (during which time the film of liquid in the pipet will continue to drain down), touch the tip of the pipet to the edge of the receiving vessel. Do not blow out the liquid remaining in the pipet after this procedure.

Finally, it is never proper to place your mouth on a pipet. Many solvents and chemicals are toxic or carcinogenic. In a biology lab one must also contend with pathogenic substances. Always imagine you are pipetting a sample of the AIDS virus or a terrible toxin.

Absolute Calibration of a Pipet

Determine the weight of distilled water of known temperature transferred by a pipet.

The degree to which the weights obtained in several trials agree is a check of your technique in the use of the pipet. Using the average of the weights and the temperature of the water calculate the absolute volume of the pipet. The volume delivered depends both on the surface tension and the viscosity of the liquid. Consequently, the calibration value is valid only for water or dilute aqueous solutions.

Use of a volumetric flask for solution preparation

Check the interior wall of the flask—particularly the neck—for uniform drainage with a small volume of the solvent. If necessary, re-clean the flask. A funnel is usually used to obtain quantitative transfer of the sample. If the space between the stem of the funnel and the neck of the flask is small, air may be trapped in the flask when liquid is added. The trapped air may in turn force liquid back up the neck of the flask. This can be avoided by using a funnel with a stem that extends into the bulb of the flask or by tipping a shorter stemmed funnel so that the end of the stem touches the wall of the flask at one point. A small piece of paper between the funnel and the top of the flask will hold the funnel in this cocked position.

Solids which dissolve readily in the solvent at room temperature may be added through the funnel if care is taken to wash the solid down with solvent. Solvent is added until the bulb of the flask is about 9/10 filled and uniform solution is obtained by swinging the flask in a small circle to promote swirling of the liquid without bringing it into the neck. Mixing at this time allows volume changes which accompany dilution to take place before the solution is made up to volume. Solvent is now added to bring the solution to the calibration mark. The last few drops may be added with a dropper. The stoppered flask is repeatedly inverted to obtain uniform mixing—at least 15 inversions, more if the solution is viscous.

Volumetric flasks should never be placed on a flame or hot plate to dissolve a difficult solute. This can cause permanent changes in the volume of the flask. If a solute is difficult to dissolve, carry out the dissolution in a beaker or flask and then quantitatively transfer the solution to the volumetric flask and bring to the final volume. Ultrasonic bath cleaners can be used to dissolve solutes in volumetric flasks.

Prepare the solution at some temperature - usually room temperature. The volume of the solution and consequently the concentration of the solution is dependent on the coefficient of expansion of the solution. (If all volumes are measured in glass equipment, then it is the difference between the coefficient for the solution and the coefficient for glass that is significant.) Around room temperature the coefficient of expansion for dilute aqueous solutions is about 0.024%/°C. A change of 4°C, therefore, corresponds to a change in concentration of about 1 ppt.

Burets

The calibration lines on a 50 ml. buret are at 0.10 ml. intervals. To obtain maximum precision, volumes are estimated to 0.01 ml. The calibrations on the 10 ml. micro-burets are at 0.020 ml. intervals and volumes are estimated to 0.002 ml.

When using a 50 ml buret, the standard deviation of a single buret reading is assumed to be ± 0.02 ml. The two readings required in measuring the volume of reagent transferred introduces an uncertainty of $[(0.02)^2 + (0.02)^2]^{1/2} = 0.03$ ml. Thus, volume less than 20 ml, even under ideal conditions, may have an uncertainty greater than 1 ppt. Most operators prefer to work in the 40 ml. range.

Use of a buret to carry out a titration

Teflon stopcocks are commonly used in burets. The Teflon stopcock requires no lubricant.

All stopcock burets are designed to be operated with the left hand so that the right hand is free to agitate the reaction mixture. With the scale of the buret facing the operator, the handle of the stopcock is on the operator's right. With the base of the left hand to the left of the buret, the thumb and first two fingers encircle the buret to control the handle of the plug, the last two fingers against the left of the tip. This braced position of the hand leads to maximum control of the stopcock. It also makes it possible to keep constant pull on the plug into a secure position in the seat. This is essential with glass stopcocks to avoid leakage. If initially the position of the left hand seems awkward, make a sensible effort to develop skill.

To fill the 50 ml buret rinse three times with 3–4 ml portions of the liquid to be used. Use a buret funnel so this liquid can be directed to flow over the entire interior surface. Do this in the buret stand to prevent any titrant which may spill from running down to your hand. Allow time for each portion to drain from the buret before the next is added. Fill the buret, including the tip, and replace the buret funnel with a buret cap. Never leave the buret funnel in the buret during a titration since it may add a drop of titrant during the titration.

Caution

If titrant is spilled on the outside of the buret, it must be cleaned up and the waste neutralized and disposed of in a proper manner.

To proceed with the titration bring the level of the liquid of the filled buret onto the scale and read the position after allowing a short time for the film of liquid to drain down the walls. The reading is more objective if an effort is not made to set the level at zero on the scale.

Using the right hand to swirl the flask and the left hand to control the stopcock, add liquid at a rapid and uniform rate. Reaction in the localized region of mixing produces an indicator change. The addition of the titrant is periodically stopped and the rapidity with which the indicator returns to its color in the first solution is observed. Using this as a guide, the addition of the titrant is continued at a gradually decreasing rate. The tip of the buret and the walls of the flask are washed down with a small volume of solvent from the wash bottle. The process of addition and rinsing is continued until the end has been located within a drop or within a fraction of a drop. After a suitable drainage period the buret is read.

Fractional drops are obtained by stopping the addition before a full drop has formed.

This fractional drop is then washed into the reaction mixture. The volume of solvent added must be adequate to bring all of the reagents into the reaction mixture at the endpoint. Premature washing with large volumes of solvent may reduce the precision of the work. This is particularly true when the concentration of the titrant is small. "Small" cannot be specified since it depends upon the properties of the reactants and the indicator. The time that should be allowed for drainage depends upon the volume of liquid withdrawn, the rate of withdrawal and the dimensions of the buret. The fine tip has been designed to place a maximum limit on the second.

The micro burets are particularly troublesome since the surface area is large in comparison to the volume. A check on the reading after a short time indicates whether adequate drainage time had been allowed.

An overrun endpoint is an overrun endpoint. In spite of this, the initial addition should be continuous and reasonably rapid. There is a limit to how long attention can be focused on drop by drop addition. If the effort invested in a sample is not large, it is good to use one sample to find the approximate volume of titrant per unit of sample taken. The estimated volume of titrant for the following samples can then be approached rapidly with confidence. Very close to the endpoint, it is good to keep a running record of buret readings (use the back side of the notebook page). This locates the endpoint between two successive readings and places a limit on the maximum error that could be involved in locating the endpoint.

Visual indicators

The selection of an indicator may be a tricky business which depends upon knowing a great deal about the chemical reactions involved. Once an indicator has been selected some familiarity with that indicator should be acquired before making a serious attempt to carry out a titration. This can be done in a very qualitative manner—even to add the titrant with a dropper to an approximate small sample in a beaker. Knowledge of the colors involved leads to confidence and greatly reduces the time consumed in the first titrations. If a back titration is feasible, the preliminary investigation provides an opportunity to decide which color change is preferred—color A to color B or color B to color A. It is easier to titrate to a definite color change but in some cases a suitable indicator is not available and it is necessary to match a color standard. The preliminary investigation sets up this color standard and gives experience in judging how rapidly the color changes. Work with an indicator until you are confident you can judge its behavior.

Determination of an indicator blank

The indicator gives the "endpoint", the point at which the titration is ended. Ideally, this would be at the "equivalence point", the point at which chemically equivalent quantities of reagents have been brought together. In practice, the endpoint and the equivalence point may not coincide. The determination of an indicator blank gives some information on this point. Even when the indicator has been correctly chosen, a significant quantity of the titrant may be required to produce the indicator change or to react with contaminants in the reagents. In some cases, it is possible to determine the quantity so used by running a blank—a titration that is equivalent in every way with the exception that the substance to be determined is not included in the reaction mixture. In order to determine an indicator blank that has meaning, the operator must be secure in their knowledge of the behavior of the indicator.

1

Acid–Base Titrations

Introduction

Titration is a common method of determining the amount or concentration of an unknown substance. The method is easy to use if the quantitative relationship between two reacting solutions is known. The acid–base titrations involve the acid–base reaction. The acid donates a proton to the base. The acid–base reactions are also known as neutralization reactions.

Acid + base $\longrightarrow$ salt + water

Acid A + base B $\longrightarrow$ conjugate acid of base B + conjugate base of acid A (Lowry-Bronsted theory)

$H^+ + OH^- \longrightarrow H_2O$ is the most general neutralization reaction

Equivalence point is the point at which the moles of H^+ are equal to the moles of OH^-. An indicator is used to show the equivalence point during a titration. A titration involves the progressive addition of one reactant from a burette (usually the acid), to a known volume of the other reactant in a conical flask (usually the base).

Calculations

a. Write the balanced chemical equation for the reaction.
b. Extract all the relevant information from the question.
c. Check that data for consistency, for example, concentrations are usually given in M or mol L^{-1} but volumes are often given in ml. You need to convert the ml to L for consistency. The easiest way to do this is to multiply the volume in ml $\times 10^{-3}$.
d. Calculate the moles of reactant (n) for which you have both the volume (V) and concentration (M) : $n = M \times V$.
e. From the balanced chemical equation find the mole ratio known reactant : unknown reactant.
f. Use the mole ratio to calculate the moles of the unknown reactant.
g. From the volume (V) of unknown reactant and its previously calculated moles (n), calculate its concentration (M) : $M = n \div V$.

Examples

1. 30 ml of 0.10 M NaOH neutralised with 25.0 ml of hydrochloric acid. Determine the concentration of the acid:
   a. Write the balanced chemical equation for the reaction:

$$NaOH \ (aq) + HCl \ (aq) \longrightarrow NaCl \ (aq) + H_2O \ (l)$$

9

b. Extract the relevant information from the question:

NaOH: $V = 30$ ml, $M = 0.10$ M; **HCl:** $V = 25.0$ ml, $M = ?$

c. Check the data for consistency

NaOH: $V = 30 \times 10^{-3}$ L, $M = 0.10$ M   **HCl:** $V = 25.0 \times 10^{-3}$ L, $M = ?$

d. Calculate moles NaOH

$$n(NaOH) = M \times V = 0.10 \times 30 \times 10^{-3} = 3 \times 10^{-3} \text{ moles}$$

e. From the balanced chemical equation find the mole ratio:

$$\begin{array}{ccc} NaOH & : & HCl \\ 1 & : & 1 \end{array}$$

f. Find moles HCl

$$\begin{array}{ccc} NaOH & : & HCl \\ 1 & : & 1 \end{array}$$

So $n(NaOH) = n(HCl) = 3 \times 10^{-3}$ moles at the equivalence point.

g. Calculate concentration of HCl : $M = n \div V$

$$n = 3 \times 10^{-3} \text{ mol}, \quad V = 25.0 \times 10^{-3} \text{ L}$$
$$M \text{ (HCl)} = 3 \times 10^{-3} \div 25.0 \times 10^{-3} = 0.12 \text{ M or } 0.12 \text{ mol L}^{-1}$$

2. 50 ml of 0.2 mol L^{-1} NaOH neutralised with 20 ml of sulfuric acid. Determine the concentration of the sulfuric acid:

a. Write the balanced chemical equation for the reaction:

$$2NaOH \text{ (aq)} + H_2SO_4 \text{ (aq)} \longrightarrow Na_2SO_4 \text{ (aq)} + 2H_2O \text{ (l)}$$

b. Extract the relevant information from the question:

NaOH: $V = 50$ ml, $M = 0.2$M;   **H$_2$SO$_4$:** $V = 20$ ml, $M = ?$

c. Check the data for consistency:

NaOH: $V = 50 \times 10^{-3}$ L, $M = 0.2$ M;   **H$_2$SO$_4$:** $V = 20 \times 10^{-3}$ L, $M = ?$

d. Calculate moles NaOH.

$$n(NaOH) = M \times V = 0.2 \times 50 \times 10^{-3} = 0.01 \text{ mol}$$

e. From the balanced chemical equation find the mole ratio

$$\begin{array}{ccc} NaOH & : & H_2SO_4 \\ 2 & : & 1 \end{array}$$

f. Find moles H$_2$SO$_4$

The equation indicates that 2 mole of NaOH is equivalent to 1 mole of: H_2SO_4

So $n(H_2SO_4) = \frac{1}{2} \times n(NaOH) = \frac{1}{2} \times 0.01 = 5 \times 10^{-3}$ moles H_2SO_4 at the equivalence point.

g. Calculate concentration of H$_2$SO$_4$: $M = n \div V$

$$n = 5 \times 10^{-3} \text{ mol}, \quad V = 20 \times 10^{-3} \text{ L}$$
$$M(H_2SO_4) = 5 \times 10^{-3} \div 20 \times 10^{-3} = 0.25 \text{ M or } 0.25 \text{ mol L}^{-1}$$

Comparison of acid and base

Theory	*Acid*	*Base*
1. Arrhenius	Proton donor	Hydroxide ion donor
2. Lowry-Bronsted	Proton donor	Proton acceptor
3. Lewis	Electron pair acceptor	Electron pair donor

EXPERIMENT 1

Determination of percentage purity of sodium bicarbonate

Sodium bicarbonate is a white solid that is crystalline but often appears as a fine powder. Sodium bicarbonate is used as an antacid to treat heartburn, indigestion, and other stomach disorders. It is also used to treat various kidney disorders and to increase the effectiveness of sulfonamides.

Experimental overview

It contains not less than 99.0% and not more than 101.0% w/w of $NaHCO_3$ calculated with reference to the dried substance.

Sodium bicarbonate is basic in nature, so titrated against standard hydrochloric acid by using methyl orange as indicator. It is a direct titration method. The equivalence point of this titration is at about pH 3.6, which lies in pH range of methyl orange (pH 2.8–4). The pink color appears at the endpoint. The reaction medium at equivalence point is acidic because of presence of carbonic acid. **Methyl orange** is used as indicator because phenolphthalein is affected by carbonic acid.

$$HCl + 2NaHCO_3 \longrightarrow 2NaCl + H_2O + CO_2$$
$$\text{Sodium bicarbonate}$$

Reagents required

1. 1 M HCl solution. Fill the volumetric flask approximately 75% full with water by using a funnel. Add the 85 ml of hydrochloric acid to the volumetric flask. Carefully, rinse any residual hydrochloric acid from the graduated cylinder and the funnel into the volumetric flask using three 5 ml portions of distilled water from a wash bottle. Stopper the volumetric flask and gently shake the solution. Fill the volumetric flask to the 1000 ml mark. Stopper the flask and gently shake the solution. If necessary, adjust the volume of the solution to 1000 ml using distilled water, and shake again.

   For preparing 1 litre of 1 M HCl solution, you need 1 mole of HCl, means 36.5 g of pure HCl. Now 36.5 divided by density 1.18 is 30.93 ml of hypothetically pure HCl, but actually it comes as a 36.5% solution, so 30.93 × 100/36.5 = 84.7 ml.

   Note: When diluting the hydrochloric acid, remember to add the concentrated acid to water to avoid splattering. Take care in handling the container as the dilution will generate heat.

2. Methyl orange indicator.
3. Anhydrous sodium carbonate.

Procedure

1. **Standardization of 1 M hydrochloric acid:**
   (i) Weigh accurately about 1.5 g of anhydrous sodium carbonate, previously heated at about 250°C for 1 hour.
   (ii) Dissolve in 100 ml of water; add 0.1 ml of methyl orange solution. Add the acid slowly from the burette with constant stirring until the solution becomes faintly pink.
   (iii) Heat the solution to boiling, cool and continue the titration. Heat again to boiling and titrate further as necessary until the faint pink color is no longer affected by continuous boiling.

Note: The reaction between sodium carbonate and hydrochloric acid takes place in two stages:

$$Na_2CO_3 + HCl \longrightarrow NaHCO_3 + NaCl \qquad \qquad ...(1)$$

$$NaHCO_3 + HCl \longrightarrow NaCl + CO_2 + H_2O \qquad \qquad ...(2)$$

In reacting with the acid, the sodium bicarbonate neutralizes it, and the pH becomes less acid. When all the acid reacts with bicarbonate, the pH ought to be neutral because salt will not affect the pH in any way (it does not form hydrogen ions). Methyl orange changes color when the pH is neutral and this indicates enough HCl solution has been added to neutralize the Na_2CO_3.

2. **Determination of sodium bicarbonate:** Weigh accurately about 1.5 g, dissolve in 50 ml of carbon dioxide free water, and titrate slowly with 1 M HCl using a further 0.2 ml of dilute methyl orange solution as indicator.

Observation and calculation

Sample calculation

1. Standardization of 1 M HCl solution

S. No.	Weight of Na_2CO_3 taken	Volume of HCl consumed	Average
1	1.5 g	15.8 ml	15.65 ml
2	1.5 g	15.5 ml	

Molecular weight of $Na_2CO_3 = 106$.

The standardization is based on the reaction of carbonate and HCl.

$$Na_2CO_3 + 2HCl \longrightarrow H_2CO_3 + 2NaCl$$

The HCl molarity is obtained from the following relation.

$$M \ HCl = \frac{\text{moles HCl}}{\text{litre}} = \frac{\text{moles of } Na_2CO_3 \times 2}{(\text{ml HCl}/1000)}$$

The factor 2 is required because each mole of Na_2CO_3 reacts with 2 moles of HCl.

$$\text{Molarity of HCl} = \frac{\text{wt. of } Na_2CO_3 \times 2}{\text{mol. wt. of } Na_2CO_3 \times \text{volume of HCl (in litre)}}$$

$$= \frac{1.5 \times 2}{106 \times 0.01565}$$

$$= 1.09 \ M$$

Alternatively, 1 M solution of sodium carbonate can be prepared by dissolving 106 g in 1000 ml of water. For determining the molarity of HCl, 20 ml of this solution is titrated with the prepared hydrochloric acid solution, using methyl orange indicator as done in previous method. From the formula, $M_1V_1 = M_2V_2$, the molarity of HCl solution can be calculated

$$M_2 = \frac{M_1V_1}{V_2}$$

where

M_1 = molarity of Na_2CO_3 solution (here, it is 1.0 M)

V_1 = volume of Na_2CO_3 solution (in flask) (here, it is 20 ml)

M_2 = ?, molarity of HCl solution

V_2 = burette volume

2. Determination of NaHCO₃

S. No.	Weight of Na₂CO₃ taken	Volume of HCl consumed	Average
1	1.5 g	19.8 ml	20.0 ml
2	1.5 g	20.2 ml	

1 mole of $NaHCO_3$ = 1 HCl

1000 ml of 1 M HCl solution = 1 M HCl = 1 M $NaHCO_3$

Mol. wt. of $NaHCO_3$ = 84

1 ml of 1.0 M HCl = 0.084 g of $NaHCO_3$

$$\text{Percentage purity} = \frac{\text{Burette reading} \times 0.084 \times \text{Molarity (cal)} \times 100}{\text{Weight of sample} \times 1.0 \, (\text{molarity known})}$$

$$= \frac{20.0 \times 0.08401 \times 1.09 \times 100}{1.5 \times 1.0} = 100.8\%$$

Result

The percentage purity of the sample was found to be 100.8%.

Judge yourself

1. What is common name for sodium bicarbonate?
2. Which indicator is used in sodium bicarbonate titration?
3. What is use of sodium bicarbonate?
4. What does "standardization of HCl solution" mean?
5. Why phenolphthalein is not used as indicator in bicarbonate titration with acid?
6. What is the pH range of methyl orange indicator?

EXPERIMENT 2

Determination of percentage purity of ammonium chloride

Ammonium chloride (NH_4Cl) is a white water-soluble crystalline salt of ammonia. The aqueous ammonium chloride solution is mildly acidic. Ammonium chloride is used as expectorant, diuretic and systemic acidifier.

Experimental overview

It contains not less than 99.0% and not more than 100.5% of NH_4Cl, calculated with reference to the dried substance.

The assay is based on indirect acid–base titration. An aqueous solution of the substance is treated with neutralized formaldehyde solution. This results in the liberation of hydrochloric acid equivalent to ammonium chloride. This is then titrated with a standard solution of sodium hydroxide using phenolphthalein as an indicator yielding pink color at the endpoint.

$$4NH_4Cl + 4H_2O \longrightarrow 4\ NH_4OH + 4\ HCl$$
$$4NH_4OH + 6\ HCHO \longrightarrow (CH_2)_6N_4 + 10H_2O$$
$$\text{(Hexamine)}$$
$$4HCl + 4NaOH \longrightarrow 4\ NaCl + 4H_2O$$

Reagents required

1. Potassium hydrogen phthalate
2. 0.1 M NaOH solution. Dissolve 4.2 g of sodium hydroxide in sufficient carbon dioxide free water to produce 1000 ml to produce 0.1 M solution.
   Note: NaOH is not a primary standard due to its hydroscopic nature.
3. Phenolphthalein indicator.

Procedure

1. **Standardization of 0.1 M sodium hydroxide solution:**
   (i) Weigh accurately about 0.5 g of potassium hydrogen phthalate (KHP), previously powdered and dried at 120°C for 2 hours, and dissolve in 75 ml of carbon dioxide free water.

Potassium acid phthalate
Molar mass 204.23 g/mol

   (ii) Add 0.1 ml of phenolphthalein solution and titrate with sodium hydroxide solution until a permanent pink color is produced.

KHP + NaOH

+H$_2$O

Sodium potassium phthalate

2. Determination of ammonium chloride:

(i) Weigh accurately about 0.1 g, dissolve in 20 ml of water, and add a mixture of 5 ml of formaldehyde solution, previously neutralized to phenolphthalein solution, and 20 ml of water.

(ii) After 2 minutes, titrate slowly with 0.1 M sodium hydroxide using a further 0.2 ml of dilute phenolphthalein solution as indicator.

Observation and calculation

Sample calculation

1. **Standardization of 0.1 M NaOH solution:**

S. No.	Weight of KHP taken	Vol. of NaOH consumed	Average vol of NaOH
1	0.5 g	20.8 ml	20.4 ml
2	0.5 g	20.0 ml	

$$\text{Molarity of NaOH} = \frac{\text{Weight of KHP (g)}}{\text{Mol. wt. of KHP} \times \text{Volume of HCl (in litre)}}$$

$$= \frac{0.5}{204 \times 0.0204} = 0.12\,M$$

Note: Each ml of 0.1 M sodium hydroxide is equivalent to 0.02042 g of $C_8H_5KO_4$.

2. **Determination of ammonium chloride:** From the equation:

$$4NH_4Cl = 4HCl = 4NaOH$$

1000 ml of 1 M NaOH solution = 1 M NaOH = 1 M NH_4Cl = 53.49 g NH_4Cl

Each ml of 0.1 M sodium hydroxide solution is equivalent to 0.005349 g of NH_4Cl

S. No.	Weight of ammonium chloride sample taken	Vol. of NaOH consumed	Average vol of NaOH consumed
1	0.1 g	14.9 ml	14.55 ml
2	0.1 g	14.2 ml	

$$\text{Percentage purity} = \frac{\text{Burette reading} \times 0.0053 \times \text{Molarity (cal)} \times 100}{\text{Weight of sample} \times \text{Molarity (given)}}$$

$$= \frac{14.55 \times 0.005349 \times 0.12 \times 100}{0.1 \times 0.1} = 93.33\%$$

Result

The percentage purity of the sample was found to be 93.33%.

Judge yourself

1. Which method was official for the assay of NH_4Cl in IP 1966?
2. What is common name for ammonium chloride?
3. Why formaldehyde is added in this titration?
4. Why formaldehyde solution is neutralized?
5. How sample of ammonium chloride is dried?
6. What is the nature of ammonium chloride salt—acidic or basic?

EXPERIMENT 3

Determination of percentage purity of borax

Borax, also known as **sodium borate**, **sodium tetraborate**, or **disodium tetraborate**, is an important boron compound. It is a salt of boric acid. It is usually a white powder consisting of soft colorless crystals that dissolve easily in water.

Borax has a wide variety of uses. It is a component of many detergents, cosmetics, and enamel glazes. It is also used to make buffer solutions in biochemistry, as a fire retardant, as an anti-fungal compound for fiberglass, as an insecticide, as a flux in metallurgy, and as a precursor for other boron compounds. It has external uses as an eyewash. It has also been used as a topical for wounds and injuries.

Experimental overview

It contains not less than 99.0% and not more than 103.0% w/w of $Na_2B_4O_7.10H_2O$. It is **basic** in nature. Hence, it is assayed by acid–base titration. On titration with hydrochloric acid, boric acid is formed. The color changes when all the boric acid has been set free. Boric acid has a very low ionization and has no effect on indicators. Methyl red changes its color in the range of 4.2–6.3 and hence, is not affected by free boric acid.

$$2HCl + Na_2B_4O_7 + 5\ H_2O \longrightarrow 2\ NaCl + 4H_3BO_3$$
$$\text{Borax} \qquad\qquad\qquad \text{Boric acid}$$

Reagents required

1. 0.5 M HCl solution. Add 45 ml of HCl solution to 100 ml of water. Make up the volume to 1 litre with water (also see page no. 12).
2. Methyl red indicator.
3. Anhydrous sodium carbonate.
4. Borax.

Procedure

1. **Standardization of 0.5 M HCl solution:**
    (i) Weigh accurately about 1.5 g of anhydrous sodium carbonate, previously heated at about 250°C for 1 hour.
    (ii) Dissolve in 100 ml of water; add 0.1 ml of methyl red solution. Add the acid slowly from the burette with constant stirring until the solution becomes faintly pink.
    (iii) Heat the solution to boiling, cool and continue the titration. Heat again to boiling and titrate further as necessary until the faint pink color is no longer affected by continuous boiling.
2. **Determination of borax:** Weigh accurately about 3 g, dissolve in 75 ml of water, and titrate slowly with 0.5 M HCl using methyl red solution as indicator (**endpoint: yellow to red**).

Observation and calculation

Sample calculation

1. **Standardisation of 0.5 M HCl:**

S. No.	Weight of Na_2CO_3 taken	Vol. of HCl consumed	Average vol of HCl consumed
1	1.08 g	30 ml	30 ml
2	1.08 g	30 ml	

$$\text{Molarity of HCl} = \frac{\text{Weight of } Na_2CO_3 \text{ (g)} \times 2}{\text{Mol. wt. of } Na_2CO_3 \times \text{Volume of HCl (in litre)}}$$

$$= \frac{1.08 \times 2}{106 \times 0.030}$$

$$= 0.6 \text{ M}$$

2. **Determination of borax:** From the reaction:

$$2HCl = Na_2B_4O_7$$

$$\text{Molecular weight of } Na_2B_4O_7.10H_2O = 381.37$$

$$1000 \text{ ml of 0.5 M HCl solution contain} = \frac{1}{2} HCl \sim \frac{1}{4} Na_2B_4O_7.10H_2O$$

Each ml of 0.5 M hydrochloric acid solution = 0.09536 g of $Na_2B_4O_7.10H_2O$

S. No.	Weight of borax sample taken	Vol. of HCl consumed	Average vol of HCl consumed
1	3 g	31.2 ml	31.35 ml
2	3 g	31.5 ml	

$$\text{Percentage purity} = \frac{\text{Burette reading} \times 0.09536 \times \text{Molarity (cal)} \times 100}{\text{Weight of sample} \times \text{Molarity (given)}}$$

$$= \frac{31.35 \times 0.09536 \times 0.6 \times 100}{3 \times 0.5} = 95.66\%$$

Result

The percentage purity of the sample was found to be 95.66%.

Judge yourself

1. What is common name of borax?
2. Give the principle involved in titration of borax.
3. What indicator is used in this titration?
4. Mention the uses of borax.
5. What do you mean by percentage purity?

EXPERIMENT 4

Determination of % purity of sodium carbonate

Sodium carbonate (also known as **washing soda** or **soda ash**), Na_2CO_3, is a sodium salt of carbonic acid. It most commonly occurs as a crystalline heptahydrate, which readily effloresces to form a white powder, the monohydrate. It has a cooling alkaline taste. It is used as electrolyte replenisher and systemic alkaliser.

Experimental overview

It contains not less than 99% and not more than the equivalent of 105.0% w/w of $Na_2CO_3.10H_2O$.

Aqueous solution of sodium carbonate is alkaline in nature. Hence, it is assayed by titrating with a standard acid using bromophenol blue as indicator. At the endpoint, an acidic pH is obtained due to the formation of carbonic acid from carbon dioxide. Hence, bromophenol blue is a indicator of choice as it shows color change in acidic range. The pH range of bromophenol blue is 2.8–4.6. Blue color is changed into yellow color at the endpoint.

$$Na_2CO_3 + H_2SO_4 \longrightarrow Na_2SO_4 + H_2O + CO_2$$

Reagents required

1. 0.5 M H_2SO_4 solution. Pour 400 ml of distilled water into a 500 ml volumetric flask. Measure 15.0 ml of H_2SO_4 in a glass graduated cylinder and carefully add to the water. Rinse graduated cylinder with water, and adjust volume to 500 ml with distilled water. Mix carefully by inversion. Store the solution in a 500 ml glass bottle.

   For preparation, first consider the molecular weight of H_2SO_4 = 98 g/mol, then you have to add 49 g of acid and make up to 1 liter of water to prepare 0.5 M sulfuric acid solution. Considering that acid is a liquid, you should consider density where density = mass/volume, but you should know density from the bottle (about 1.84 g/L) then you have:

   $$\text{volume} = 49/1.84 = 26.60 \text{ ml}$$

   Now you have to consider the acid purity, usually 98% then you have to do this:

   $$\frac{26.60 \times 100}{98} = 27.15 \text{ ml}$$

   Then you have to measure 27.15 ~ 30 ml of sulfuric acid 98% and make it up to 1 liter with distilled water.

   Note: Add the sulfuric acid slowly to avoid the splattering. Take care in handling as the dilution will generate heat.

2. Bromophenol blue indicator.
3. Anhydrous sodium carbonate.
4. Methyl orange indicator.

Procedure

1. **Standardization of 0.5 M H_2SO_4 solution:** Weight out about 1.3 g of anhydrous sodium carbonate accurately using the method of "weighing by difference". Transfer the weighed

carbonate to a beaker and add about 100 ml of distilled water to dissolve it completely. Add 2 drops of methyl orange indicator. Titrate the carbonate solution with the given dilute sulfuric acid until the color of solution just changes from yellow to orange. Repeat the titration twice.

Each ml of 0.5 M H_2SO_4 solution = 0.05299 g or 52.99 mg of Na_2CO_3

2. **Determination of sodium carbonate:** Weigh accurately about 0.5 g, dissolve in 20 ml of water, and titrate with 0.5 M sulfuric acid solution, using bromophenol blue solution as indicator till yellow color appears (**endpoint: blue to yellow**).

Observation and calculation

1. **Standardization of sulfuric acid:** The standardization of sulfuric acid is based on the reaction of sulfuric acid with sodium carbonate:

$$H_2SO_4 + Na_2CO_3 \longrightarrow H_2CO_3 + Na_2CO_3$$

$$\text{Molarity of sulfuric acid} = \frac{\text{Weight of } Na_2CO_3 \text{ (g)}}{106 \times \text{Vol. of } H_2SO_4 \text{ consumed (in litre)}}$$

106 is the molecular weight of anhydrous Na_2CO_3.

2. **Determination of sodium carbonate:** From the equation:

$$1 \text{ mole of } Na_2CO_3 = 1 \text{ mole of } H_2SO_4$$

Molecular weight of $Na_2CO_3.10H_2O$ = 286

1000 ml of 0.5 M H_2SO_4 solution contain $\frac{1}{2} H_2SO_4$ equivalent to $\frac{1}{2} Na_2CO_3.10H_2O$

Each ml of 0.5 M sulfuric acid solution is equivalent to 0.143 g of $Na_2CO_3.10H_2O$

S. No.	Weight of sodium carbonate sample taken	Vol. of H_2SO_4 consumed	Average vol of H_2SO_4 consumed
1	0.5 g	ml	'M' ml
2	0.5 g	ml	

$$\text{Percentage purity} = \frac{\text{Burette reading} \times 0.143 \times \text{Molarity (cal)} \times 100}{0.5 \times 0.5 \text{ (given molarity)}}$$

Result

The percentage purity of the sample was found to be ... %.

Judge yourself

1. What is common name for sodium carbonate?
2. How the equivalent weight of sodium carbonate is calculated?
3. What is the pH range for methyl orange and methyl red indicator?
4. What is the meaning of "weighing by difference"?
5. Suggest one method other than using acid–base indicator to detect the endpoint of an acid–alkali titration.
6. How anhydrous sodium carbonate is prepared?

EXPERIMENT 5

Determination of aspirin using back titration

Aspirin is in a group of drugs called salicylates. It works by reducing the synthesis of substances (prostaglandins) in the body that cause pain, fever, and inflammation. Aspirin is used to treat mild to moderate pain, and also to reduce fever or inflammation. It is sometimes used to treat or prevent heart attacks, strokes, and angina.

Experimental overview

Many reactions are slow or present unfavorable equilibria for direct titration. Aspirin is a weak acid that also undergoes slow hydrolysis; i.e. each aspirin molecule reacts with two hydroxide ions. To overcome this problem, a known excess amount of base is added to the sample solution and an HCl titration is carried out to determine the amount of unreacted base. This is subtracted from the initial amount of base to find the amount of base that actually reacted with the aspirin and hence the quantity of aspirin in the analyte.

Reagents required

1. 0.1 M HCl solution. Add 8.5 ml of HCl solution to 100 ml of water. Make up the volume to 1 litre with water (*also see page no. 12*).
2. 0.1 M NaOH solution. Dissolve 4.2 g of NaOH in 1000 ml of water. *See page no. 15 for its standardization*. Take 0.9 to 1.0 g of anhydrous sodium carbonate and follow the same procedure.
3. Aspirin.
4. Phenolphthalein indicator.
5. Phenol red indicator.

Procedure

Determination of aspirin in powder

1. Accurately weigh three samples of 0.40–0.45 g each into 150 ml Erlenmeyer flasks. Do not dry the samples, Dissolve each sample in turn in 15 ml of alcohol, add 4 drops phenolphthalein indicator, and titrate each sample quickly to the first persistent faint pink color with standard 0.1 M NaOH solution.
2. Record this volume. Then add, from your buret, that same volume again + 5 ml excess. Place the flasks on the steam bath for 45 minutes to allow reaction (2) to proceed to completion. Then, back-titrate the excess base with your standard 0.1 M HCl solution.

Determination of aspirin content in tablet (IP method)

1. Weigh accurately 20 tablets and find out the average weight of tablet. Powder them.
2. Weigh accurately powder equivalent to 0.5 g of aspirin.
3. Add 30 ml of 0.5 M sodium hydroxide solution.
4. Heat the mixture on a water bath gently for 10 minutes. Cool down the mixture and titrate the excess of alkali with 0.1 M HCl solution using phenol red solution as indicator.
5. Similarly, perform the blank titration.

Observation and calculation

Determination of aspirin in powder

Sample calculation

Weight of aspirin sample: 0.3828 g.

Volume of 0.1 M NaOH solution used for neutralization: 18.89 ml.

Volume of total 0.1056 M NaOH solution was added for complete hydrolysis and neutralization: 42.78 ml (18.89 + 18.89 + 5 ml = 42.78 ml).

Volume of 0.1056 M HCl solution used during back titration: 14.29 ml.

First recognize that the 18.89 ml of base was used to neutralize all acidic material present in the sample. Since we are only interested in the quantity of acetylsalicylic acid, we must determine the quantity of base required for neutralisation of acidic material and hydrolysis of the ester (here 2 mole of NaOH is equivalent to 1 mole of aspirin).

Total number of moles of base added is:
$$\text{moles NaOH} = 0.04278 \text{ L} \times 0.1000 \text{ M} = 4.278 \times 10^{-3} \text{ mol}$$

The number of moles of HCl used in the titration corresponds to the excess NaOH, or the number of moles not consumed in the hydrolysis reaction:
$$\text{moles HCl} = \text{moles excess NaOH}$$
$$= 0.1056 \text{ M} \times 0.01429 \text{ L}$$
$$= 1.509 \times 10^{-3} \text{ mol}$$

The difference between the number of moles of total base added and those which were not consumed equals the number of moles of base that brought about hydrolysis and neutralisation. This is related to the number of moles of acetylsalicylic acid:
$$4.278 \times 10^{-3} - 1.509 \times 10^{-3} = 2.769 \times 10^{-3} \text{ mol}$$
$$\text{Moles of aspirin} = \frac{2.769 \times 10^{-3}}{2} = 1.3845 \times 10^{-3}$$

The number of grams acetylsalicylic acid is found using the molecular weight of acetylsalicylic acid:
$$\text{g (of aspirin)} = 2.769 \times 10^{-3} \text{ mol} \times 180.2 \text{ g/mol}$$
$$= 0.2492 \text{ g acetylsalicylic acid}$$

Thus, % purity $= \dfrac{0.2492}{0.3828} \times 100 = 65\%$.

Note: Here 18.89 ml (required for neutralisation) or 18.89 + 5.0 ml = 23.89 ml of 0.1 M NaOH can also be correlated with moles of aspirin. Here, 1 mole of 0.1 M NaOH is equal to 1 mole of aspirin.

Result

The % purity of aspirin sample is = 97.25%.

Determination of aspirin content in tablet

Volume of 0.5 M NaOH added = 30 ml.

Moles of NaOH = $0.030 \times 0.5 = 1.5 \times 10^{-3}$.

Suppose, volume of 0.5 M HCl required to react with excess of unreacted 0.5 M NaOH solution is 10 ml.

Moles of HCl = Moles of excess of NaOH = $0.010 \times 0.50 = 0.5 \times 10^{-3}$.

Moles of NaOH which reacted with aspirin:

$$1.5 \times 10^{-3} - 0.5 \times 10^{-3} = 1.0 \times 10^{-3} \text{ or } \frac{1.0 \times 10^{-3}}{2} \text{ moles of aspirin}$$

Mass of aspirin = $1.0 \times 10^{-3} \times 180 = 0.180$ g of aspirin

Thus, the content of aspirin/average wt. tablet $= \dfrac{0.180}{\text{Weight of powder}} \times$ average wt of tablet.

Alternative method (IP method)

The content of aspirin can also be determined by using the factor in a usual way.

The sample (aspirin powder—1.5 g) is heated under refluxing condition with 50 ml of 0.1 M NaOH solution for 10 minutes. Cool down and titrate with 0.1 M HCl solution by using phenol red as indicator. Similarly, perform the blank titration.

Each ml of 0.1 M NaOH solution = 0.090 g of aspirin.

Weight of powder = W g

Average weight of tablet = Z g

Volume of 0.1 M NaOH solution which reacted with aspirin

$\qquad$ = (blank reading – sample reading) = V ml

Molarity of NaOH = M

The content of aspirin/average wt. tablet $= \dfrac{0.090 \times V \times M \text{ (cal)}}{W \times 0.1} \times Z = \dots$ g of aspirin.

Judge yourself

1. Why aspirin is estimated by back titration?
2. Why alcohol is added in the assay of aspirin?
3. What are the different uses of aspirin?
4. Why did you use your burette and not a graduated cylinder to add the excess of NaOH solution?
5. Which indicator is used in the assay of aspirin?
6. What is difference between Erlenmeyer and volumetric flasks?
7. Why did you use burette and not a graduated cylinder to add excess NaOH?

EXPERIMENT 6

Determination of the percentage purity of given sample of boric acid

Boric acid (H_3BO_3), also called **boracic acid** or **orthoboric acid**, is a weak acid. It is used as an antiseptic, insecticide, flame retardant, in nuclear power plants to control the fission rate of uranium, and as a precursor of other chemical compounds. It exists in the form of colorless crystals or a white powder and dissolves in water.

Experimental overview

Boric acid contains not less than 99.5 and not more than 100.5%.

This assay is based on acid–base type of titration. Boric acid, which is a very weak acid, is difficult to titrate against strong alkali like sodium hydroxide. However, by addition of certain organic polyhydroxy compound such as mannitol, sorbitol or glycol, it acts as strong acid and can be titrated with strong base by using phenolphthalein indicator.

The effect of polyhydroxy compound can be explained on the basis of formation of 1:1 and 1:2 ratio complexes between hydrated and borate ion on 1, 2 or 1, 3–diols.

Boric acid is esterified in the presence of glycerin producing a strong glyceroborate complex which can act as strong acid. The mannitol and sorbitol are more effective. As they are solid in nature, these are required in small quantity and they do not change volume of titrant.

Reagents required

1. Boric acid.
2. Potassium hydrogen phthalate (KHP).
3. 0.1 M sodium hydroxide solution. Dissolve about 4.2 g of NaOH in 1 litre of distilled water.
4. Glycerin.
5. Phenolphthalein indicator.

Procedure

1. **Standardization of 0.1 M sodium hydroxide:** Accurately mass approx. 0.2 g of KHP into a 250 ml Erlenmeyer flask. Add about 100 ml of water and swirl the flask until the sample is dissolved. Add 3 drops of phenolphthalein indicator (colorless in acidic solution; pink in basic solution). Titrate the KHP solution with the base solution to be standardized. Titration should proceed until the faintest pink persists for 30 sec. after swirling. The color will fade upon exposure to the air. Make duplicate determinations and calculate the average molarity of the NaOH. For excellent work, the molarities need to be within 1% of one another.

2. **Assay of boric acid:**
    (a) Weigh accurately about 0.8 g of sample acid, add 10 ml of water and 10 ml of glycerol previously neutralized to phenolphthalein solution and dissolve the sample completely.
    (b) To this mixture add few drop of phenolphthalein as indicator. Titrate with 0.1 M NaOH until color change from colorless to pink.
    (c) Report the burette reading three times. Record the average volume 'V' ml.

Observation and calculation

Determination of molarity of NaOH

$$\text{Molarity of NaOH} = \frac{\text{Weight of KHP (g)}}{204 \times \text{Volume of NaOH (in litre)}}$$

where 204 is the molecular weight of KHP.

Determination of boric acid

Factor

$H_3BO_3 + NaOH \longrightarrow NaBO_2 + 2 H_2O$
Molecular weight of boric acid = 61.84
1 M of H_3BO_3 = 1M NaOH = 1000 ml of 1 M NaOH
61.84 gm of H_3BO_3 = 1000 ml of 1 M NaOH
0.00618 gm of H_3BO_3 = 1 ml of 0.1 M of NaOH
The weight of boric acid sample taken: W g
The volume of NaOH solution consumed = V ml

$$\text{The } V \text{ ml of 0.1 M NaOH solution} = \frac{V \times 0.00618 \times \text{Molarity (cal)}}{0.1 \,(\text{Molarity given})} \text{ g of } H_3BO_3$$

$$\text{The } W \text{ g of boric acid contain} = \frac{V \times 0.00618 \times M}{0.1} \text{ g of } H_3BO_3$$

$$\% \text{ purity of boric acid} = \frac{V \times 0.00618 \times \text{Molarity (cal)}}{0.1 \,(\text{Molarity given}) \times W} \times 100 = \dots \%.$$

Result

The given sample of boric acid contains ... % w/w of H_3BO_3.

Judge yourself

1. Why glycerin is added in the boric acid determination?
2. Mention the standards of boric acid according to IP 2007?
3. What is the uses of boric acid?
4. Why glycerin is neutralized?
5. What is the reaction of mannitol with boric acid?

EXPERIMENT 7

Volumetric determination of carbonate and bicarbonate in a mixture

Experimental overview

The main challenge in this experiment is that we need to quantitatively determine both HCO_3^- or CO_3^- and then one of the components alone. The remaining constituent then can be calculated by subtraction of the one component from total alkalinity determination

A titration of your sample directly with strong acid will lead to reactions with both carbonate and bicarbonate in stoichiometric proportions (see relevant reactions). The sum of all acid moles or equivalents used is a useful piece of information called total alkalinity for the mixture of carbonate and bicarbonate.

Reactions

Strong acid with bicarbonate: $HCO_3^- + H^+ \longrightarrow H_2CO_3$

Strong acid with carbonate: $CO_3^{2-} + 2H^+ \longrightarrow H_2CO_3$

Strong base with bicarbonate: $HCO_3^- + OH^- \longrightarrow CO_3^{2-} + H_2O$

Precipitation of carbonate with barium: $Ba^{2+} + CO_3^{2-} \longrightarrow BaCO_3 \, (s)$

Strong acid with strong base: $H^+ + OH^- \longrightarrow H_2O$

But, how can we measure HCO_3^- or CO_3^- using volumetric methods? One approach might be to titrate with strong base to determine HCO_3^- however, the endpoint will be difficult to determine. Thus, our measurement challenge would be simplified if we could remove or isolate the bicarbonate from the carbonate. But this cannot be done easily or conveniently. Both of these complications can be solved using the method of excess reagent and back-titration with strong reagents. What is a back–titration? In a back–titration, an exact and excess amount of strong base is added to solution to react with HCO_3^- (there will be no reaction between OH^- and CO_3^-) and some OH^- will remain as residual base in solution. We may arrange a clean back-titration of residual OH^- with strong acid when all forms of carbonate are removed from the sample. This can be accomplished when a soluble barium salt is added to the solution before a titration is attempted, carbonate will be precipitated as $BaCO_3$ and will be eliminated as an interference. Thus, determination consists of:

a. Determination of all HCO_3^- and CO_3^- using a strong acid titration.

b. Determination of HCO_3^- using back-titration with strong acid of excess OH^- after eliminating CO_3^- (from original sodium carbonate and from the reacted bicarbonate) by precipitation as $BaCO_3$ from the solution.

Reagents required

1. 0.1 M HCl solution. Dissolve 8.5 ml of HCl solution in 100 ml of water. Make up the volume to 1 litre. (*Please also see page no.* 12).

2. 0.1 M NaOH solution. Dissolve about 4.2 g of NaOH in 1 litre of distilled water.

3. 10% w/v $BaCl_2$ solution.

4. Phenolphthalein indicator.

5. Methyl red indicator.

6. Bromocresol green indicator.

Procedure

A. Standardization of 0.1 M HCl solutions

1. Dry primary standard-grade sodium carbonate for 1 hour at 110°C and cool it in a desiccator. Bring to constant weight. Weigh approximately containing enough Na_2CO_3 to react with ~25 ml of 0.1 M HCl and place each in a 250 ml flask. Add 25 ml of distilled water, swirl the flask to dissolve the solid and add 3 drops of methyl red indicator solution. Titrate one rapidly to a pink color to find an approximate endpoint. The stoichiometry of the reaction is shown here:

$$2HCl + Na_2CO_3 \longrightarrow CO_2 + 2NaCl$$

2. Titrate carefully other samples to the pink color endpoint. During each titration, you should periodically tilt and rotate the flask to wash all liquid from the walls into the bulk solution using deionized water from a plastic squeeze bottle. When very near the end, you should deliver less than 1 drop of titrant at a time.

3. Calculate the mean HCl molarity.

$$\text{Molarity of HCl} = \frac{\text{Wt. of } Na_2CO_3 \,(g) \times 2}{\text{Mol. wt. of } Na_2CO_3 \times \text{Volume of HCl (in litre)}}$$

B. Preparation and standardization of 0.1 M NaOH solution

All NaOH solutions come with impurities and contamination the make each NaOH solution imprecise unless calibrated. Calibrated NaOH solutions have limited shelf-life even when protected against atmospheric carbon dioxide. Furthermore, store your solution only in a plastic bottle and insure that the cap is free of solution between uses.

1. Place (using a volumetric pipette) 25.00 ml of your dilute HCl solution into a 250 ml Erlenmeyer flask. Add 2–3 drops of phenolphthalein indicator solution, and titrate to an endpoint with the NaOH solution. The endpoint is the first appearance of faint pink color that persists for 15 seconds (The color will slowly fade as CO_2 from the air dissolves in the solution.)

2. Make two more replicate determinations of 25.00 ml of NaOH solution using the standardized HCl solution. Calculate the average molarity with the formula, M_1V_1 (HCl) $= M_2V_2$ (NaOH).

C. Volumetric determination of carbonate and bicarbonate

1. Store Solid unknown in a desiccator to keep dry; however, do not heat the sample. Even mild heating at 50°–100°C converts $NaHCO_3$ to Na_2CO_3. Accurately, weigh 2.0 to 2.5 g of unknown into a clean 250 ml volumetric flask. A funnel may be used to aid transfer of sample to the volumetric flask. Rinse the funnel repeatedly with small portions of freshly boiled and cooled water to dissolve and transfer the sample to the flask. Remove the funnel, mix well, and dilute to the mark. This is your unknown solution.

2. Pipette a 25.00 ml aliquot of the unknown solution into a 250 ml Erlenmeyer flask, add 3 drops of bromocresol green indicator solution and titrate rapidly (to a green endpoint) using your standardized HCl solution (from above). Then, repeat in triplicate this procedure carefully with 25.00 ml samples of unknown solution. Record the average titre value 'M' ml. This volume will give us total alkalinity.

3. Pipette a 25.00 ml aliquot of the unknown solution and 50.00 ml of your standardized NaOH solution into a 250 ml flask. Swirl thoroughly and add using a graduated cylinder 10 ml of 10% w/w $BaCl_2$ solution. Swirl again to precipitate $BaCO_3$, add 2 drops of phenolphthalein

indicator, and immediately titrate (the endpoint is a faint pink) with your standardized HCl solution. Do all of this quickly without delay.

4. Repeat in triplicate this procedure carefully with 25.00 ml samples of your unknown solution. Record the average titre value 'N' ml.

5. Calculate the total alkalinity in the unknown solution and calculate the bicarbonate concentration in the unknown solution. Based upon volumetric amounts and dilution volumes, calculate % of sodium carbonate and percent sodium bicarbonate in your solid sample.

Observation and calculation

Weight of sample = W g

Volume of 0.1 M HCl solution consumed by total alkali (CO_3^{2-} and HCO_3^-) = M ml

Volume of 0.1 M HCl solution consumed in back titration = N ml

Suppose molarity of HCl and NaOH solution is same

Then, the volume of NaOH solution reacted with HCO_3^- = 50 – N = 'O' ml

Volume of HCl equivalent to 'O' ml of NaOH solution or equivalent to HCO_3^- = O ml (as molarity is same)

Volume of 0.1 M HCl solution consumed by CO_3^{2-} = $M - O = P$ ml

Calculation for NaHCO$_3$: From the equation:

NaHCO$_3$ = HCl = 1000 ml of 1 MHCl

Molecular weight of NaHCO$_3$ = 84

Each ml of 0.1 M HCl solution = 0.0084 g of NaHCO$_3$

'O' ml of 0.1M HCl solution = 0.0084 × 'O' g of NaHCO$_3$

25 ml of sample solution contain = 0.0084 × 'O' g of NaHCO$_3$

250 ml solution or W g sample contain = 0.0084 × O × 10 g of NaHCO$_3$

$$\% \text{ of NaHCO}_3 = \frac{0.0084 \times O \times 10 \times 100}{W} \text{ g of NaHCO}_3$$

Calculate for Na$_2$CO$_3$: From the equation:

Na$_2$CO$_3$ = 2HCl = 2000 ml of 1 M HCl

Molecular weight of Na$_2$CO$_3$ = 106

Each ml of 0.1 M HCl solution = 0.0053 g of Na$_2$CO$_3$

'P' ml of 0.1 M HCl solution = 0.0053 × P g of Na$_2$CO$_3$

25 ml of sample solution contain = 0.0053 × P g of Na$_2$CO$_3$

250 ml solution or W g sample contain = 0.0053 × P × 10 g of Na$_2$CO$_3$

$$\% \text{ of Na}_2\text{CO}_3 = \frac{0.0053 \times P \times 10 \times 100}{W} \text{ g of Na}_2\text{CO}_3$$

Result

The % of sodium carbonate = … w/w%.

The % of sodium bicarbonate = … w/w%.

Judge yourself

1. Why solid sample is not heated to constant weight while primary standard is heated to constant weight?
2. Why tap water instead of de-ionized water in preparing solutions is used?
3. What happen if barium precipitation step is forgotten?
4. Why it is advised to store your solutions in plastic bottle not glass containers.
5. What do you mean by total alkalinity of water?

EXPERIMENT 8

Determination of ibuprofen using acid/base titration

Ibuprofen, 2–(p-isobutyl phenyl propanoic acid, $(CH_3)_2CHCH_2 C_6H_4CH(CH_3)COOH$ is a well known nonsteroidal anti-inflammatory (NSAID), analgesic and antipyretic agent.

Experimental overview

Ibuprofen when dried contains not less than 98.5% $C_{13}H_{18}O_2$. It has acidic character due to presence of free carboxylic group. Hence, it is determined by titration with base.

Reaction

Ibuprofen   Sodium salt of Ibuprofen

Reagents required

1. 0.1 M NaOH solution. Dissolve about 4.2 g of NaOH in 1000 ml of distilled water.
2. Potassium hydrogen phthalate.
3. Phenolphthalein indicator.
4. Ibuprofen.

Procedure

A) Determination of ibuprofen in powder sample

1. **Standardization of 0.1 M NaOH solution:** The NaOH solution will be your titrant. Rinse a buret with water and then with a small amount of the NaOH solution. Fill the buret with NaOH solution. Accurately weigh about 0.5 g of KHP into a 250 ml Erlenmeyer flask. Add about 100 ml of water and swirl the flask until the sample is dissolved. Add 3 drops of phenolphthalein indicator (colorless in acidic solution; pink in basic solution). Titrate the KHP solution with the base solution to be standardized. Titration should proceed until the faintest pink persists for 30 sec. after swirling. Calculate the molarity of NaOH solution as in Experiment 1.
2. **Determination of ibuprofen in powder:**
   (i) Weigh accurately about 400 mg of ibuprofen drug sample and dissolve in 100 ml of ethanol (95%).
   (ii) Titrated with 0.1 M sodium hydroxide solution using 0.2 ml of phenolphthalein solution as indicator.
   (iii) Perform blank determination and make necessary correction to calculate the drug content.

B) Determination of ibuprofen in tablet

1. Weigh accurately 20 tablets and find out the average weight of tablet. Powder them.
2. Weigh accurately the powder equivalent to 0.5 g of ibuprofen, extract with 60 ml of chloroform and filter.

3. Wash the residue with quantities of chloroform (3 × 25 ml) and gently evaporate the filtrate to dryness.
4. Dissolve the residue in 100 ml of alcohol and titrate with 0.1 M sodium hydroxide solution using 0.2 ml of phenolphthalein solution as indicator.
5. Perform blank determination and make necessary correction to calculate the drug content.

Observation and calculation

A. **Standardization of 0.1 M NaOH solution:**

$$\text{Molarity (M) of NaOH} = \frac{\text{Weight of KHP (g)}}{204 \times \text{Vol. of NaOH consumed (in litre)}}$$

B. **Determination of Ibuprofen in powder sample:** From the equation:

Volume consumed in blank titration = V_1 ml

Volume of 0.1 M NaOH solution consumed in sample titration = V_2 ml

Actual volume of 0.1 M NaOH reacted with ibuprofen = $V_2 - V_1 = V$ ml

1 mole of ibuprofen = 1 mole of NaOH

Molecular weight of Ibuprofen = 206.28

Each ml of 0.1 M NaOH solution = 0.020628 g of $C_{13}H_{18}O_2$

$$\% \text{ purity of Ibuprofen} = \frac{0.020628 \times V \times M \text{ (cal)}}{W \times 0.1 \text{ (molarity given)}} \times 100 = ...\%$$

C. **Determination of ibuprofen in tablet:**

Each ml of 0.1 M NaOH = 0.020628 g of $C_{13}H_{18}O_2$

Weight of powder = W g

The average weight of tablet = Z g

The volume of 0.1 M NaOH consumed = V ml (difference of sample and blank titration)

The Molarity of NaOH = M

$$\text{The content of ibuprofen / average wt. tablet} = \frac{0.020628 \times V \times M \text{ (cal)}}{W \times 0.1} \times Z = ...\text{g of ibuprofen}$$

Judge yourself

1. How ibuprofen acts as anti-inflammatory drug?
2. Why NaOH is not a primary standard?
3. Mention the various primary standard used to standardize NaOH.
4. What does "standardization of NaOH solution" mean?
5. Why tablet powder is extracted with chloroform?

EXPERIMENT 9

Determination of percentage purity of indomethacin by acid–base titration

Indomethacin is a non-steroidal anti-inflammatory indole derivative designated chemically as 1-(4-chlorobenzoyl)-5-methoxy-2-methyl-1H-indole-3-acetic acid. Indomethacin is practically insoluble in water and sparingly soluble in alcohol. It has a pKa of 4.5 and is stable in neutral or slightly acidic media and decomposes in strong alkali. The suspension has a pH of 4.0–5.0. The structural formula is:

Indomethacin

Experimental overview

Indomethacin contain not less than 90.0% and not more than 110% of stated amount of indomethacin, $C_{19}H_{10}ClNO_4$. It has acidic character due to presence of free carboxylic group. Hence, it is determined by titration with base.

Reaction

Indomethacin	Sodium salt of Indomethacin

Reagents required

1. 0.01 M NaOH solution. Dissolve 0.42 g in 1 litre of water.
2. Potassium hydrogen phthalate.
3. Phenolphthalein indicator.

Procedure

1. **Standardization of 0.01 M NaOH.** Please see page no. 24.
2. **Determination of indomethacin:** Dissolve about 0.025 g of indomethacin in a flask by the addition of 10 ml of neutral acetone, shake then filter into a conical flask and wash twice with 10 ml of neutral acetone. Titrate the filtrate with 0.01 M NaOH solution using phenolphthalein solution as an indicator.

Observation and calculation

For calculation of molarity of NaOH, please see page no. 25.

    1 mole of Indomethacin = 1 mole of NaOH

    Molecular weight of indomethacin = 357.3

    Each ml of 0.01 M NaOH solution = 0.003573 g of Indomethacin

$$\% \text{ purity of Indomethacin} = \frac{0.003573 \times V \times M \text{ (cal)}}{W \times 0.01} \times 100 = ...\%$$

where V is the volume of NaOH consumed.

       W = weight of sample

       M = Molarity of NaOH solution

Result

The % purity of Indomethacin is found to be ... %.

Judge yourself

    1. Why indomethacin contraindicated in elderly patients?

    2. What is dose of indomethacin?

    3. Which other method is recommended for the assay of indomethacin capsule?

    4. What are the uses of indomethacin?

EXPERIMENT 10

Determination of sodium hydroxide and sodium carbonate in a mixture

Experimental overview

Double indicator method is employed to determine NaOH and Na_2CO_3 when present together. The principle involved in this method is that when sodium carbonate is titrated with HCl, the neutralization occurs in two steps. The first one corresponds to the hydrogen carbonate (HCO_3^+) stage. The net reaction is: $CO_3^{2-} + H^+ \longrightarrow HCO_3^-$

The equivalence point for determination for the primary stage of ionization of carbonic acid is at pH 8.3 which may be detected by using phenolphthalein indicator. The second stage of the titration corresponds to displacement of all carbonic acid, when the net reaction is:

$$CO_3^{2-} + 2H^+ \longrightarrow H_2CO_3$$
$$HCO_3^- + H^+ \longrightarrow H_2CO_3$$
$$H_2CO_3 \longrightarrow H_2O + CO_2$$

The equivalence point for the secondary stage of ionization is at pH 3.1–4.4 which may be detected by employing methyl orange indicator. Then, when a mixture of Na_2CO_3 and NaOH is titrated with standard HCl, the phenolphthalein endpoint corresponds to the neutralization of all NaOH and all neutralization of all the Na_2CO_3 to the bicarbonate stage.

$$NaOH + HCl \longrightarrow NaCl + H_2O$$
$$Na_2CO_3 + HCl \longrightarrow NaCl + NaHCO_3$$

Now if the titration is continued using methyl orange as indicator, the neutralization of the bicarbonate to the carbonic acid occurs.

$$NaHCO_3 + HCl \longrightarrow NaCl + H_2CO_3$$
$$H_2CO_3 \longrightarrow H_2O + CO_2$$

So that methyl orange endpoint means the total volume of acid run down from the beginning of the experiment.

Thus if the titre value $\{P\}$ and $\{M\}$ corresponds to the phenolphthalein and methyl orange endpoint, the:

$$\{P\} = NaOH + \tfrac{1}{2}Na_2CO_3$$
$$\{M\} = NaOH + Na_2CO_3$$
$$\{M\} - \{P\} = \tfrac{1}{2}Na_2CO_3$$
$$2[\{M\}\ ] - \{P\}] = Na_2CO_3$$
$$\{M\} - 2[\{M\}\ ] - \{P\}] = NaOH$$

Reagents required

1. 0.1 N HCl solution. Add 8.5 ml of HCl to few ml of distilled water. Mix and volume is make up to 1 litre in volumetric flask.
2. Phenolphthalein indicator.
3. Methyl orange indicator.

Procedure

1. Pipet out 10 ml of alkali mixture into 250 ml conical flask. Add 2–3 drops of Phenolphthalein indicator.

2. Titrate with 0.1 N HCl solution from burette until the solution becomes colorless. Note the titre value [P] ml.
3. Then, add 2–3 drops of methyl orange indicator and continue the titration until red color is obtained. Note the titre value [M] ml.

Observation and calculation

No.	Vol of alkali mixture	Phenolphthalein indicator vol of HCl consumed (P)	Methyl orange indicator vof HCl consumed (M)
1.	10 ml	–	–
2.	10 ml	–	–
3.	10 ml	–	–

NaOH content

Equivalent weight of NaOH = 40

1000 ml of 1 N HCl solution = 40 g of NaOH

1 ml of 0.1 N HCl solution = 0.004 g of NaOH

$\{M\}-2(M-P)$ ml of 0.1 N HCl solution = $0.004 \times [\{M\} -2 (M-P)]$ g of NaOH

The quantity of NaOH(g)/litre = $\dfrac{0.004 \times [\{M\} - 2(M-P)] \times 1000}{10}$ g of NaOH = 'X' g/litre

Na$_2$CO$_3$ content

Equivalent weight of Na$_2$CO$_3$ = 53

1000 ml of 1 N HCl solution = 53 g of NaOH

1 ml of 0.1 N HCl solution = 0.0053 g of Na$_2$CO$_3$

2 $(M-P)$ ml of 0.1 N HCl solution = $0.0053 \times 2 (M-P)$ g of Na$_2$CO$_3$

The quantity of Na$_2$CO$_3$(g)/litre = $\dfrac{0.0053 \times 2(M-P)] \times 1000}{10}$ g of Na$_2$CO$_3$ = 'Y' g/litre

Result

The given alkali mixture contains
= 'X' g/litre of NaOH
= 'Y' g/litre Na$_2$CO$_3$

Judge yourself

1. What do you mean by total alkalinity of water?
2. What is difference between endpoint and equivalence point.
3. Calculate the equivalent weight of sodium carbonate and sodium bicarbonate.
4. What is the color of methyl orange in acid and basic medium?
5. What is the chemical formula for: (i) Caustic soda, (ii) Washing soda.
6. How the color of phenolphthalein and methyl orange changes?

EXPERIMENT 11

Determination of % purity of zinc oxide

Zinc oxide is an inorganic compound with the formula, ZnO. It usually appears as a white powder, nearly insoluble in water. The powder is widely used as an additive into numerous materials and products including plastics, ceramics, glass, cement, rubber (e.g. car tyres), lubricants, paints, ointments, adhesives, sealants, pigments, foods (source of Zn nutrient), batteries, ferrites, fire retardants, etc.

Experimental overview

Zinc oxide contains not less than 99% and not more than the equivalent of 100.5% w/w of ZnO, calculated with reference to the ignited substance.

It is back titrated due to slow reaction between zinc oxide and sulfuric acid. Excess of standard sulfuric acid is added and unreacted acid is back titrated with standard sodium hydroxide solution. Ammonium chloride is added to prevent the precipitation of zinc hydroxide both during the titration and also at the endpoint. The precipitation of zinc hydroxide would give poor endpoint.

$$ZnO + H_2SO_4 \longrightarrow ZnSO_4 + H_2O$$
$$H_2SO_4 + 2NaOH \longrightarrow Na_2SO_4 + 2H_2O$$

Reagents required

1. 0.5 M H_2SO_4 solution. Pour 400 ml of distilled water into a 500 ml volumetric flask. Measure 15.0 ml of H_2SO_4 in a glass graduated cylinder and carefully add to the water. Rinse graduated cylinder with water, and adjust volume to 500 ml with distilled water. Mix carefully by inversion. Store the solution in a 500 ml glass bottle (please also see Experiment 4).

2. 0.5 M NaOH solution. Dissolve about 2.1 g in 1 litre of distilled water.

3. Methyl orange indicator.

Procedure

1. **Standardization of 0.5 M H_2SO_4 solution:** Weight about 1.0 g of anhydrous sodium carbonate accurately using the method of "weighing by difference". Transfer the weighed carbonate to a 250 ml flask and add about 100 ml of distilled water to dissolve it completely. Add 2 drops of methyl orange indicator. Titrate the carbonate solution with the given dilute sulfuric acid until the color of solution just changes from yellow to orange. Repeat the titration two times.

   Each ml of 0.5 M H_2SO_4 solution = 0.05299 g or 52.99 mg of Na_2CO_3

2. **Determination of Zinc oxide:** Dissolve an accurately weighed quantity of zinc oxide (about 1.5 g) and 2.5 g of ammonium chloride in 50 ml of 0.5 M sulfuric acid solution with the aid of gentle heating. Add few drops of methyl orange as indicator and titrate the solution with 0.5 M sodium hydroxide solution till yellow color appears.

Observation and calculation

A. Standardization of sulfuric acid

$$\text{Molarity of sulfuric acid} = \frac{\text{Weight of } Na_2CO_3 \text{ (g)}}{106 \times \text{Vol. of } H_2SO_4 \text{ consumed (in litre)}}$$

B. Determination of ZnO

Molecular weight of ZnO = 81.41

Weight of sample = W g

Volume of 0.5 M NaOH consumed by unreacted sulfuric acid = M ml

Suppose molarity of NaOH and H_2SO_4 is same.

Volume of 0.5 M H_2SO_4 reacted with ZnO = 50 – M = V ml

From the equation:

1 mole of ZnO = 1 mole of H_2SO_4 = 1000 ml of 1 M H_2SO_4 solution

Each ml of 0.5 M H_2SO_4 solution = 0.04068 gm of ZnO.

$$\text{The \% purity of ZnO} = \frac{0.020628 \times V \times \text{Molarity (cal)}}{W \times 0.5\,(\text{molarity given})} \times 100 = ...\%$$

Result

The % purity of zinc oxide is = ... %.

Judge yourself

1. Why ZnO is assayed by back titration?
2. Why ammonium chloride is added in this back titration?
3. What is need of standardizing the sulfuric acid?
4. What are the uses of ZnO?
5. Name the other volumetric method for the assay of zinc oxide.

EXPERIMENT 12

Determination of % purity of lactic acid

Lactic acid (2–hydroxypropanoic acid), also known as **milk acid**, is a chemical compound that plays a role in several biochemical processes. It was first isolated in 1780 by a Swedish chemist, Carl Wilhelm Scheele, and is a carboxylic acid with a chemical formula of $C_3H_6O_3$. It has a hydroxyl group adjacent to the carboxyl group, making it an alpha hydroxy acid. In solution, it can lose a proton from the acidic group, producing the **lactate** ion $CH_3CH (OH)COO^-$. It is miscible with water or ethanol, and is hygroscopic.

Lactic acid is chiral and has two optical isomers. One is known as *L*-(+)-lactic acid or *(S)*-lactic acid and the other, its mirror image, is *D*-(-)-lactic acid or *(R)*-lactic acid. *L*-(+)-Lactic acid is the biologically important isomer.

Experimental overview

Lactic acid consists of mixture of lactic acid, lactoyl lactic acid and various other condensation polymers derived from it. In the assay procedure, both lactic acid and condensation products are determined. Hydrolysis of lactoyl lactic acid and other condensation products with excess of NaOH produces lactic acid which together with free lactic acid is neutralized by NaOH solution. The excess of sodium hydroxide is back titrated with standard HCl solution.

$$CH_3CHOHCOOH + NaOH \longrightarrow CH_3CHOHCOONa + H_2O$$

Lactic acid Sodium lactate

$$CH_3CHOHCOO + H_2O + 2NaOH \longrightarrow 2CH_3CHOHCOONa$$

$$|$$

$$CH_3CHCOOH$$

Sodium lactate

Lactoyl-lactic acid

Reagents required

1. 0.1 M HCl solution. Dissolve 8.5 ml of concentrated HCl solution in 750 ml of water in volumetric flask. Shake and make up the volume (Please also see Experiment 1).
2. 0.1 M NaOH solution. Dissolve 4.2 g of NaOH in 1 litre of water.
3. Phenolphthalein indicator.

Procedure

1. Standardization of 0.1 M NaOH solution (see Experiment 2).
2. Standardization of 0.1 M HCl solution (see Experiment 1).
3. Determination of lactic acid:
   (i) Weigh accurately about 0.2 g of lactic acid in weighing bottle and transfer into conical flask with the help of water.
   (ii) Add accurately measured 50 ml of 0.1 M NaOH solution nd allow to stand for 30 minutes.
   (iii) Titrate the excess of NaOH solution with 0.1M HCl solution using phenolphthalein indicator.

Observation and calculation

Molecular weight of lactic acid = 90.08

Weight of sample = *W* g.

Volume of 0.1 M HCl consumed by unreacted NaOH solution = M ml.

Suppose molarity of NaOH and HCl is same.

Volume of 0.1 M NaOH reacted with lactic acid = $50 - M = V$ ml

From the equation:

1 mole of $CH_3CHOHCOOH$ = 1 mole of NaOH = 1000 ml of 1 M NaOH solution.

Each ml of 0.1 M NaOH solution = 0.009008 g of $CH_3CHOHCOOH$

$$\text{The \% purity of lactic acid} = \frac{0.009008 \times V \times \text{Molarity (cal)}}{W \times 0.1 \,(\text{molarity given})} \times 100 = ... \%$$

Result

The % purity of lactic acid is = ... %.

Judge yourself

1. Why lactic acid is assayed by back titration?
2. What are the uses of lactic acid?
3. Why lactic acid is called milk acid?
4. What is chiral carbon? Show its presence in structure of lactic acid.
5. What is qualitative test for lactic acid?

EXPERIMENT 13

Determination of % purity of sodium benzoate

Sodium benzoate is the sodium salt of benzoic acid. One gram of the salt is soluble in 2 ml of water, in 75 ml of ethyl alcohol, and in 50 ml of 90% ethyl alcohol. The salt is insoluble in ethyl ether.

Sodium benzoate is widely used as chemical preservative in carbonated and still beverages, syrups, olives, sauces, relishes, jellies, jams and pastry low fat salad dressing, fruit salads, prepared salads, and in storage of vegetables.

Experimental overview

It is a basic compound due to liberation of sodium hydroxide on hydrolysis. The liberated sodium hydroxide reacts with standard hydrochloric acid. Ether is added to solubilize the benzoic acid.

$$C_6H_5COONa + HCl \longrightarrow C_6H_5COOH + NaCl$$
$$\text{Sodium benzoate} \qquad \text{Benzoic acid}$$

Reagents required

1. 0.5 M HCl solution. Dissolve about 45 ml of HCl solution into water and make up the volume to 1 litre.
2. Ether.
3. Bromophenol blue indicator.

Procedure

1. **Standardization of 0.5M HCl solution:**
   (i) Weight out about 1.3 g of anhydrous sodium carbonate accurately using the method of "weighing by difference".
   (ii) Transfer the weighed carbonate to a beaker and add about 100 ml of distilled water to dissolve it completely. After dissolving, transfer the solution to a 250 ml volumetric flask. Rinse the beaker thoroughly and transfer all the washes into the volumetric flask. Remember not to overshoot the graduation mark of the flask. Make up the solution to the mark on the neck by adding water.
   (iii) Pipette 25.00 ml of sodium carbonate solution to a clean conical flask. Add 2 drops of methyl orange indicator to the carbonate solution.
   (iv) Titrate the carbonate solution with the given dilute hydrochloric acid until the color of solution just changes from yellow to orange.
   (v) Repeat the titration two times.
   (vi) Calculate the molarity (please see Experiment 1).
2. **Determination of Sodium benzoate:** Weigh accurately about 1.5 g of sodium benzoate, previously dried and transfer into a 250 ml flask with a ground–glass stopper. Dissolve in 25 ml of water, add 75 ml of ether and 2–3 drops of bromophenol blue indicator. Titrate with 0.5 M hydrochloric acid titration while mixing the water and ether layers well by shaking until a light green color persists in the water layer.

Observation and calculation

Molecular weight of sodium benzoate = 142

Weight of sample = W g

Volume of 0.5 M HCl consumed = V ml

From the equation:

1 mole of C_6H_5COONa = 1 mole of HCl = 1000 ml of 1 M HCl solution

Each ml of 0.5 M HCl solution = 0.07205 g of $C_7H_5NaO_2$

$$\text{The \% purity of sodium benzoate} = \frac{0.072005 \times V \times \text{Molarity (cal)}}{W \times 0.5 \, (\text{molarity given})} \times 100 = \dots \%$$

Result

The % purity of sodium benzoate is = ... %.

Judge yourself

1. What is basis of its estimation?
2. What are the uses of sodium benzoate?
3. How sodium benzoate acts as preservative?
4. What is the pH of bromophenol blue indicator?
5. Why ether is added in sodium benzoate titration?

EXPERIMENT 14

Determination of % purity of Sodium phosphate

Sodium phosphate ($Na_2HPO_4.12H_2O$) is a sodium salt of phosphoric acid. It is a white powder that is highly hygroscopic and water soluble. It is therefore used commercially as an anti-caking additive in powdered products. It is also known as disodium hydrogen orthophosphate, sodium hydrogen phosphate or sodium phosphate dibasic. It is commercially available in both the hydrated and anhydrous forms. Disodium phosphate can be used in cream of wheat to quicken cook time, as described on the ingredients panel of the product package.

Experimental overview

Sodium phosphate contains not less than 99% and not more than 101.0% with reference to substance dried to constant weight at 130°C.

It is titrated with standard hydrochloric acid by using bromocresol green indicator. On reaction with HCl sodium phosphate produces Sodium dihydrogen phosphate.

$$Na_2HPO_4 + HCl \longrightarrow NaH_2PO_4 + NaCl$$
Disodium hydrogen   Sodium dihydrogen
phosphate   phosphate

Reagents required

1. 0.5 M HCl solution. Dissolve about 45 ml of HCl solution into water and make up the volume to 1 litre.
2. Bromocresol green color.
3. Sodium phosphate

Procedure

1. **Standardization of 0.5M HCl solution:**
   (i) Weight out about 1.2 g of anhydrous sodium carbonate accurately using the method of "weighing by difference".
   (ii) Transfer the weighed carbonate to a beaker and add about 100 ml of distilled water to dissolve it completely. After dissolving, transfer the solution to a 250 ml volumetric flask. Rinse the beaker thoroughly and transfer all the washes into the volumetric flask. Remember not to overshoot the graduation mark of the flask. Make up the solution to the mark on the neck by adding water.
   (iii) Pipette 25.00 ml of sodium carbonate solution to a clean conical flask. Add 2 drops of methyl orange indicator to the carbonate solution.
   (iv) Titrate the carbonate solution with the given dilute hydrochloric acid until the color of solution just changes from yellow to orange.
   (v) Repeat the titration two times.
   (vi) Calculate the molarity (see Experiment 1).

2. **Determination of Sodium phosphate:**
   (i) Weigh accurately about 1.5 g of sodium phosphate and dissolve in 100 ml of water.
   (ii) Add few drops of bromocresol green indicator and titrate with 0.5 HCl solution until green color appears.

Observation and calculation

Weight of sample = W g

Volume of 0.5 M HCl consumed = V ml

From the equation:

1 mole of Na_2HPO_4 = 1 mole of HCl = 1000 ml of 1 M HCl solution

Each ml of 0.5 M HCl solution = 0.01791 g of Na_2HPO_4

$$\text{The \% purity of sodium phosphate} = \frac{0.01791 \times V \times \text{Molarity (cal)}}{W \times 0.5 \,(\text{molarity given})} \times 100 = ... \%$$

Result

The % purity of sodium phosphate is = ... %.

Judge yourself

1. What is basis of its estimation?
2. What are the uses of sodium phosphate?
3. How do you prepare a 1 liter (L) 0.1 M HCl from a 12 M HCl solution?
4. What is the pH range of bromocresol green indicator? Mention the other indicators which can be used in this titration.

EXPERIMENT 15

Determine and compare the acid neutralizing power of two commercial antacids

Introduction

Hydrochloric acid (HCl) is one of the substances found in gastric juices secreted by the lining of the stomach. HCl is needed by the enzyme pepsin to catalyze the digestion of proteins in the food we eat. Heartburn is a symptom that results when the stomach produces too much acid (hyperacidity).

Experimental overview

Antacids are bases used to neutralize the acid that causes heartburn. Despite the many commercial brand, almost all antacids act on excess stomach acid by neutralizing it with weak bases. The most common of these bases are hydroxides, carbonates, or bicarbonates. The following table contains a list of the active ingredients found in several common commercial antacids, and the reactions by which these antacids neutralize the HCl in stomach acid.

Compound	Chemical formula	Chemical reaction
Aluminum hydroxide	$Al(OH)_3$	$Al(OH)_3 + 3HCl \rightarrow AlCl_3 + 3H_2O$
Calcium carbonate	$CaCO_3$	$CaCO_3 + 2HCl \rightarrow CaCl_2 + H_2O + CO_2$
Magnesium carbonate	$MgCO_3$	$MgCO_3 + 2HCl \rightarrow MgCl_2 + H_2O + CO_2$
Magnesium hydroxide	$Mg(OH)_2$	$Mg(OH)_2 + 2HCl \rightarrow MgCl_2 + 2H_2O$
Sodium bicarbonate	$NaHCO_3$	$NaHCO_3 + HCl \rightarrow NaCl + H_2O + CO_2$

In this experiment, 2 brands of antacids will be analyzed to determine the number of moles of acid neutralized per tablet. The analytical procedure used is known as **back titration**.

Why back titration?

Common ingredients in antacids are metal hydroxide and metal carbonate salts. The hydroxides provide hydroxide ion, OH^-, which can react with $H^+(aq)$ to form H_2O. Carbonates provide the carbonate ion, CO_3^{2-}, which can react with $H^+(aq)$ to form H_2O and CO_2. The reactions of interest in this lab are neutralization reactions as shown below.

$$H^+ (aq) + OH^- (aq) \rightarrow H_2O$$
$$2 H^+ (aq) + CO_3^{2-} (aq) \rightarrow H_2O + CO_2 (g)$$

To determine the amount of base in an actual tablet, ideally you would dissolve it in water and titrate with acid. In most titrations, solutions of the acid and the base are used. This is not an option here because $CaCO_3$ is quite insoluble in water. By the time the tablet completely dissolves, you will have added too much acid. To overcome this problem, the antacid tablet is dissolved in a known amount of excess acid; the excess acid is neutralized with more base.

Tablet $[Mg(OH)_2/CaCO_3]$ + HCl $\rightarrow$ Neutralized tablet + excess acid $\rightarrow$ Acidic solution excess
HCl + NaOH $\rightarrow$ Neutral solution

The excess of HCl is titrated with NaOH(aq) until enough OH⁻ (from the NaOH solution) has been added to completely react with the excess H⁺ (from the excess HCl in the solution). So, part of the added acid is neutralized by the antacid tablet; the remainder is neutralized by the NaOH added. This is called back titration.

Reagents required

1. 0.5 M HCl solution
2. 0.5 M NaOH solution
3. Antacid tablets
4. Phenolphthalein indicator

Procedure

1. Standardization of 0.5 M HCl solution, see Experiment 3.
2. Standardization of 0.5 M NaOH solution, see Experiment 2.
3. Determination of neutralizing capacity of antacid tablets
   (i) Obtain an antacid tablet and grind it into a fine powder. Weigh out two samples of about 0.5 to 0.6 g of antacid powder in weighing bottle, recording the exact masses used in each trial.
   (ii) Place one sample of the antacid tablet into a clean 250 ml Erlenmeyer flask and rinse the weighing bottle using distilled water.
   (iii) Add approximately 25 ml of distilled water, and stir the solution to dissolve the antacid sample. (Note: the antacid will likely not completely dissolve.)
   (iv) Add 2 or 3 drops of phenolphthalein indicator to the solution. (Note: the solution should become light red in color.)
   (v) Clean a buret, and fill it with 0.1 M HCl solution. Add 49–50 ml HCl solution to the antacid solution, recording the exact volume used. At this point the indicator should turn colorless, and the rest of the sample should be dissolved.
   (vi) Mix the solution thoroughly, and carefully warm the mixture on a hot/stir plate. Allow the solution to gently boil for about 2 minutes. (Note: considerable bubbling will occur because of the liberation of CO_2 gas from the carbonic acid-bicarbonate system as mentioned in the discussion.

      If the pink/red color returns during/after boiling, cool the flask and add accurately measured amount of acid (1 or 2ml of acid at a time until the color disappears. Boil again for two minutes. If the solution remains colorless, proceed as follows.
   (vii) Cool the flask under cold tap water, and rinse down the inside walls of the flask with distilled water.
   (viii) Back titrate the boiled antacid/HCl solution with NaOH solution. Titrate the solution to the first permanent (~10 seconds) pink color, and record the exact volume used.

      Note: In case of bromophenol blue if used in place phenolphthalein, the color changes from yellow to blue)
   (ix) Repeat steps ii–viii with the second antacid sample.
   (x) Repeat steps i–ix with a second brand of antacid.

Data:

Molarity of HCl used: ... .
Molarity of NaOH used: ... .

	Trial 1	Trial 2	Trial 1	Trial 2
Commercial antacid (name)				
Mass of antacid (g)				
Initial volume of HCl (ml)				
Final volume of HCl (ml)				
Volume of HCl added (ml)				
mmol of HCl added				
Initial volume of NaOH (ml)				
Final volume of NaOH (ml)				
Volume of NaOH added (ml)				
mmol of NaOH added				
mmol of H^+ reacted mmol of H^+ reacted/g of antacid				
Average mmol of H^+ reacted/g of antacid				

Observation

Illustrated with following example

[HCl] = 0.100 M   Volume of HCl added = 50.00 ml
[NaOH] = 0.100 M   Volume of NaOH required = 5.00 ml

mass of antacid = 0.600 g

Calculations:

Total mole of HCl present in 50 ml of 0.1 M HCl = $50 \times 0.1/1000 = 5 \times 10^{-3}$ mole

Total mole of HCl (unreacted) present in 5 ml of 0.1 M NaOH or 0.1 M HCl = $5 \times 0.1/1000$

$\qquad = 0.5 \times 10^{-3}$ mole provided the molarility of NaOH and HCl are equal (0.1 M)

Total mole of HCl reacted (neutralized) with antacid tablet = 5×10^{-3} mole $- 0.5 \times 10^{-3}$ mole

$\qquad\qquad = 45 \times 10^{-3}$ mole

Amount of HCl neutralized by 1 gm of antacid = $45 \times 10^{-3}/0.600 = 7.5 \times 10^{-3}$ mole of HCl

Amount of HCl (gm) neutralized by 1 gm of antacid = $7.5 \times 10^{-3} \times 36.5/1$ mole

$\qquad\qquad = 0.27375$ g/per gm of antacid

Result

The neutralization capacity of antacid tablet (Brand I) = ... mole/per g of antacid or ... g/per g of antacid tablet.

The neutralization capacity of antacid tablet (Brand II) = ... mole/per g of antacid or ... g/per g of antacid tablet.

Judge yourself

1. Some commercial antacids are colored. How might this can affect our analysis?
2. From the list of active ingredients on the packets, write word equations for the reactions that take place in your flask during the titrations.
3. What is neutralizing capacity?
4. Name some brand of antacid tablets.
5. Why back titration is preferred to determine the acid neutralizing capacity?

Precipitation Titrations

Introduction

Precipitation titration as the name suggest involve the formation of precipitates. Quite commonly, chlorides are detected by the formation of white precipitates of silver chloride on adding silver nitrate solution to the soluble chloride salt. This familiar test is efficiently used for the quantitative estimation of inorganic soluble salt. For example, sodium chloride is estimated on the basis of chloride by titration with silver nitrate solution. Silver nitrate react with chloride to form the insoluble silver chloride. The endpoint can be detected by observing

   (i) Cessation of precipitation or
  (ii) Using internal indicator or
 (iii) Using instrumental methods like potentiometric or amperometric methods.

Precipitation methods are classified into:
   (a) Mohr's method
   (b) Volhard's method
   (c) Fajans method
   (d) Gay-Lussac method

(a) Mohr's method

This method is official in IP 1966 for the estimation of neutral salt like sodium chloride. Accurately weighed quantity of sodium chloride is dissolved in water, acidified with nitric acid and titrated with standard silver nitrate solution by using potassium chromate as indicator. Sodium chloride form insoluble precipitates of silver chloride on reacting with silver nitrate solution.

$$NaCl + AgNO_3 \longrightarrow AgCl + NaNO_3$$

At the endpoint when all the quantity of sodium chloride has been consumed, a slight excess of silver nitrate react with indicator, potassium chromate, to form reddish brown precipitates of silver chromate.

$$2AgNO_3 + K_2CrO_4 \longrightarrow Ag_2CrO_4 + 2KNO_3$$
$$\text{Potassium} \qquad \text{Silver}$$
$$\text{chromate} \qquad \text{chromate}$$

Note: Titration can be performed in neutral solution only as silver chromate is unstable in acidic solution.

(b) Volhard method

1. **Direct titrations:** Compounds of silver and mercury are estimated by direct titration with standard ammonium thiocyanate solution by using ferric ammonium sulfate as indicator.

$$Hg^+ + NH_4SCN \longrightarrow Hg(SCN)_2 \downarrow + NH_4^+$$
$$\text{Mercuric}$$
$$\text{thiocyanate}$$

$$Ag^+ + NH_4SCN \longrightarrow Ag(SCN) \downarrow + NH_4^+$$
$$\text{Silver}$$
$$\text{thiocyanate}$$

Silver and mercury salts form insoluble precipitate of their respective thiocyanate on reaction with standard ammonium thiocyanate solution. At the endpoint when total quantity of metal salt has been reacted, a slight excess of ammonium thiocyanate solution react with indicator to form colored precipitate of ferric thiocyanate.

$$3NH_4SCN + Fe(NH_4)(SO_4)_2 \longrightarrow Fe(SCN)_3 \downarrow + 2(NH_4)_2SO_4$$
$$\text{Ferric ammonium} \qquad\qquad \text{Ferric}$$
$$\text{sulphate} \qquad\qquad\qquad \text{thiocyanate}$$

Solution must be acidified in this titration to avoid the precipitation of silver nitrate as phosphate or carbonate and ferric alum.

Yellow mercury oxide and mild silver protein are assayed by this method in IP 1966.

2. **Indirect titrations:** Inorganic halides are quantitatively estimated by this method. For example, assay of sodium chloride is based on complete precipitation of soluble chloride as insoluble chloride in nitric acid solution by adding excess of accurately measured standard silver nitrate solution. The excess of silver nitrate is then determined by back titration with standard ammonium thiocyanate solution by using ferric ammonium sulphate as indicator.

$$NaCl + AgNO_3 \longrightarrow AgCl \downarrow + NaNO_3$$
$$AgNO_3 + NH_4SCN \longrightarrow AgSCN \downarrow + NH_4NO_3$$

Silver nitrate forms insoluble precipitate of sodium chloride on reaction with soluble sodium chloride. On titration the excess of silver nitrate reacts with ammonium thiocyanate to form insoluble precipitate of silver thiocyanate and at the endpoint, when entire quantity of silver nitrate has been reacted, a slight excess of ammonium thiocyanate reacts with indicator to form red color precipitate of ferric thiocyanate.

There are two sources of errors: (i) In the titration of silver with thiocyanate some silver nitrate may be adsorbed by the precipitate, leading to the premature endpoint. This may be avoided by vigorous shaking. (ii) Silver thiocyanate is less soluble (7.1×10^{-13}) than silver chloride (1.2×10^{-10}). So, as soon as silver has been titrated and the excess of thiocyanate is present, the equilibrium:

$$AgCl + SCN^- \rightleftharpoons AgSCN + Cl^-$$

occur, consuming thiocyanate and leading to a significant over-titration. Hence, the precipitate of silver chloride is either removed by filtration or coagulated by adding organic solvent like nitrobenzene, dibutyl phthalate. The organic solvents form a protective layer on the precipitate of silver chloride to avoid its interaction with ammonium thiocyanate.

$$AgCl + NH_4SCN \longrightarrow AgSCN \downarrow + NH_4Cl$$

(c) Fajans method

It includes the titration of halide with standard silver nitrate solution by using adsorption indicator (introduced by Fajan). The fluorescein, dichloroflurecin, eosin, etc. are the common examples of adsorption indicator. For example, chlorides are titrated with standard silver nitrate. Adsorption indicators are acidic dyes, so ionize to give their colored anion. At the equivalence point when all the chloride has been consumed, these colored anions are adsorbed to the precipitate and give their own color; means endpoint is marked by the appearance of different color.

(d) Gay-Lussac method

This method was introduced by Gay-Lussac, and is also referred as turbidity method. In this standard solution of silver chloride with the solution of silver nitrate in nitric acid or vice versa, but indicator is not added. The endpoint is marked by the cessation of precipitate formation. It means addition of silver nitrate gives the precipitation of silver nitrate. At the endpoint when all the sodium chloride will be consumed there will be no precipitate formation on addition of silver nitrate solution, a small quantity of pure barium nitrate to assist the coagulation of precipitate. It is advisable to carry out titration twice. The first titration is used to take approximate reading. In the second determination, silver nitrate is added dropwise (in about 0.05 ml portion) near the endpoint to have the exact endpoint.

EXPERIMENT 16

Determination of sodium chloride by Mohr's method

Sodium chloride, also known as **common salt**, is a chemical compound with the formula NaCl. Sodium chloride is the salt most responsible for the salinity of the ocean and of the extracellular fluid of many multicellular organisms. As the major ingredient in edible salt, it is commonly used as a condiment and food preservative.

Experimental overview

The Mohr titration uses the chromate ion as an indicator for the titration of chloride with silver nitrate solution. After the chloride is consumed, the slight excess of silver nitrate reacts with the chromate to form an orange yellow precipitate. As the indicator and analyte reactions are competitive equilibria, the concentration of the indicator must be carefully chosen. Ideally, a concentration of 6.1×10^{-3} M CrO_4^{2-} will initiate precipitation of Ag_2CrO_4 at the equivalence point of the titration. Experimentally, it has been found that 2×10^{-3} M is the optimum concentration.

$$NaCl + AgNO_3 \longrightarrow AgCl^- \downarrow + NaNO_3$$
White precipitate

$$Ag^+ + Cl^- \longrightarrow AgCl(s) \; k_{sp} = 1.8 \times 10^{-10}$$

$$2AgNO_3 + K_2CrO_4 \longrightarrow Ag_2CrO_4 \downarrow + 2KNO_3$$
Silver chromate

$$2Ag^+ + CrO_4^{2-} \longrightarrow Ag_2CrO_4(s) \; k_{sp} = 1.1 \times 10^{-12}$$

Reagents required

1. 0.1 M silver nitrate solution. Prepare approximately 0.1 M $AgNO_3$ by dissolving about 8.5 g of $AgNO_3$ in 500 ml of deionized water. Mix well and store in a dark glass bottle.
   Caution: Silver nitrate is very corrosive. It is never to be weighed on an analytical balance. It may damage the balance. It can also burn the skin, use caution. (It is also expensive—**do not waste it**).
2. 5% w/v potassium chromate indicator solution: Dissolve 1.0 g of K_2CrO_4 in 20 ml of distilled water.
3. Sodium chloride reference substance.

Procedure

1. **Standardization of 0.1 M silver nitrate solution:** Use the analytical balance to weigh out 0.75–1.0 g (weighed to the nearest 0.1 mg) of pure, dry NaCl and dissolve it in 250 ml of distilled water in a volumetric flask. Pipet 25.0 ml of this solution into a titration flask and add 4 drops of 5% w/v K_2CrO_4 solution. Titrate with the silver nitrate solution until you observe the appearance of an orange-yellow precipitate while vigorously stirring the solution. Vigorous stirring of the solution is necessary to maintain equilibrium throughout the solution. Repeat the titration at least three times.
   Each ml of 0.1 M silver nitrate solution = 0.005844 g of NaCl.
   Note: (1) Restandardise before use. (2) Discard the solution after 30 days. (3) Store in amber bottle with well-fitted suitable stoppers which prevent access to atmospheric carbon dioxide.

2. **Determination of sodium chloride:** Use the analytical balance to weigh out sodium chloride (about 0.25 gm), dissolve in water (50 ml) and titrate with 0.1 M silver nitrate solution using a 5% w/v potassium chromate as an indicator. Repeat the whole procedure.

   Note: The Mohr titration should be carried out under conditions of pH 6.5–9. At higher pH silver ions may be removed by precipitation with hydroxide ions, and at low pH chromate ions may be removed by an acid–base reaction to form hydrogen chromate ions or dichromate ions, affecting the accuracy of the endpoint.

Observation and calculation

1. Calculation of molarity of standard $AgNO_3$ solution:

$$\text{Molarity} = \frac{W\ (g)}{58.44 \times V\ \text{(in litre)}}$$

where W = Weight of sodium chloride in g

   V = Volume of silver nitrate solution consumed in litre

   58.44 = Molecular weight of NaCl

2. **Determination of sodium chloride:**

   Molecular weight of NaCl = 58.44
   Weight of the sample = W g

Determination of sodium chloride in unknown sample:

S. No.	Weight of unknown sample	Volume of AgNO₃
1	0.20 g	V ml
2	0.25 g	V ml
3	0.18 g	V ml

The volume of 0.1 M $AgNO_3$ solution consumed = V ml
From the above equation, 1 mole of NaCl = 1 mole of $AgNO_3$
Hence, 1 ml of 0.1 M $AgNO_3$ solution = 0.005844 gm of NaCl.

$$\% \text{ of sodium chloride} = \frac{0.005844 \times V \times \text{molarity (cal)}}{W \times 0.1\,(\text{molarity given})} \times 100 = \dots \%$$

Result

The percentage purity of sodium chloride sample is ... %.

Judge yourself

1. Why Mohr's method is not applied for the determination of ammonium chloride?
2. Why silver nitrate is not a primary standard?
3. How the endpoint is detected in Mohr's method?
4. What are the uses of sodium chloride?

EXPERIMENT 17

Determination of chloride by the Fajans method

Experimental overview

The Fajans method is a direct titration of chloride with silver ions (from silver nitrate) by using dichlorofluorescein (DCF) dye as the indicator:

$$Ag^+ + Cl^- \longrightarrow AgCl(s) \; Ksp = 1.8 \times 10^{-10}$$

4′,5′-Dichlorofluorescein

The indicator reaction takes place at the surface of the precipitate. The indicator is a weakly acidic dye and exists in solution in the ionized form, In^-. The titrant is a silver solution, and during the titration a precipitate of AgCl is formed. Initially, this precipitate is colloidal, consisting of very small non-settling particles with a diameter of less than 1 μm. While this would be undesirable for a gravimetric determination (colloids cannot be filtered), it is advantageous for an adsorption indicator method. What happens is the following.

Precipitates have a tendency to adsorb "their own" ions to the surface to form what is known as the primary adsorption layer, i.e. AgCl preferentially adsorbs Ag^+ or Cl^-, whichever happens to be in excess. A colloidal precipitate has a very large surface area and, therefore, presents an abundance of room for adsorption. Before the equivalence point of the titration of Cl^- with Ag^+, the Cl^- ion is in excess and forms the primary adsorption layer on the surface of the AgCl precipitate. The particles have a negative surface charge and repel each other; the colloid is stabilized by this. The indicator ion, In^-, is also repelled and stays well away from the surface. Because the particles are negatively charged, they attract cations that are in solution more strongly than anions. Thus, there is weakly-bound secondary adsorption layer consisting of the cation that forms the most insoluble chloride to AgCl (probably Na^+); these ions form the secondary adsorption layer.

Beyond the equivalence point, Ag^+ is in excess and the surface of the precipitate becomes positively charged, with the primary layer being Ag^+. These positively charged colloidal particles will now attract the indicator anion (In^-) and adsorb it into secondary adsorption layer.

The indicator forms a colored complex with silver ion, imparting a color to the precipitate. Only at the surface is the silver ion concentration high enough for the solubility product of the complex to be exceeded; this does not happen anywhere else in the solution, and the color is therefore confined to the precipitate surface.

The pH must be controlled for reliable results. If it is too low, the indicator (a weak acid) is dissociated too little to produce enough In^-.

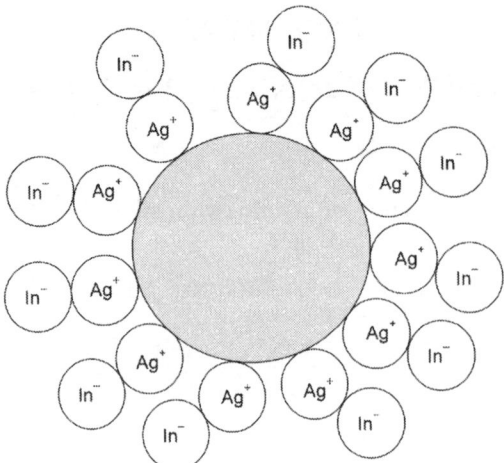

At the equivalence point, neither titrant nor titrate ions are in excess, and the precipitate is momentarily without a surface charge. This causes the colloidal particles to coagulate, thereby reducing the precipitate surface area. It can be prevented by the addition of a small amount of dextrin (hydrolyzed starch) to the solution.

The titration reaction is:

$$AgNO_3 \text{ (aq)} + NaCl \text{ (aq)} \longrightarrow AgCl \text{ (s)} + NaNO_3 \text{ (aq)}$$

In fact, because neither Na^+ nor NO_3^- ions are involved in the reaction, this reaction may be written more accurately as:

$$Ag^+ + Cl^- \equiv AgCl \text{ (s)}$$

The nitrate ions are only weakly adsorbed to the precipitate after the equivalence point is reached, and they are easily displaced by indicator ion. The **endpoint** is signaled by the appearance of the **pink color** of silver dichlorofluoresceinate.

Silver chloride is very sensitive to photodecomposition in the presence of the indicator. The titration will probably fail if attempted in direct sunlight. If this is a problem, do a trial titration and use the volume of $AgNO_3$ added as the approximate volume to reach the endpoint for the subsequent titrations. For these subsequent titrations, wait to add the indicator and dextrin until just before (a few ml the endpoint. Continue the titration without delay.

Reagents required

1. 0.1 M $AgNO_3$ solution. Prepare approximately 0.1 M $AgNO_3$ by dissolving about 8.5 g of $AgNO_3$ in 500 ml of deionized water. Mix well and store in a dark glass bottle.
2. NaCl reference substance.
3. Dichlorofluorescein indicator. Dissolve 0.2 g of dichlorofluorescein in a solution prepared by mixing 75 ml of ethanol and 25 ml of water.

Procedure

1. **Standardization of 0.1 M $AgNO_3$:** Silver nitrate is not a primary standard due to purity reasons. Hence, needs standardization.
   (i) Transfer approximately one gram of reagent grade NaCl from the container in the oven into a glass weighing bottle. Allow the NaCl to cool in a desiccator for 15 to 30 min.

(ii) Dry the unknown in an oven at 100°C for 1 hr. Allow the unknown to cool to room temperature in a desiccator. Weigh accurately about 0.15–0.20 g of the dried NaCl into 250 ml Erlenmeyer flasks. Dissolve in approximately 60 ml of deionized water.

Note: The mass of the NaCl in the solution is important, not the volume of the solution, so you can use a graduate cylinder to measure the 60 ml of water.

(iii) Add 10 drops of the indicator solution (dichlorofluorescein) and roughly 0.1 g of dextrin (no need to weigh the dextrin) to the NaCl solution.

(iv) Rinse the buret at least 3 times with a few ml of the approximately 0.1 M $AgNO_3$ solution. Fill the buret with the 0.1 M $AgNO_3$ solution and be sure to eliminate all bubbles in the tip before continuing.

(v) Immediately titrate the sodium chloride solution with silver nitrate until the first permanent appearance of the pink color of the indicator.

(vi) Calculate the average molarity of $AgNO_3$.

2. **Titration of unknown:**

(i) Weigh 0.20 to 0.29 g of the unknown sample to the nearest 0.0001 g.

(ii) Titrate the unknown sample as done for standardization of silver nitrate solution.

(iii) Repeat the titration at least two more times.

Observation and calculations

1. Calculation of molarity of standard $AgNO_3$ solution

$$\text{Molarity} = \frac{W\ (g)}{58.44 \times V(L)}$$

W = Mass of NaCl in g

V = Volume of M $AgNO_3$ solution consumed (in litre)

Mol. weight of NaCl = 58.44

2. % Cl in unknown sample

Mass of unknown sample = W_1 g

The % Cl in the unknown is calculated from the volume of $AgNO_3$ required for the titration.

$$\text{Moles Cl}^- = M_{AgNO_3} \times V_{AgNO_3}$$

$$\text{Mass Cl}^- = \text{moles Cl}^- \times \text{atomic weight of Cl}^-$$

$$\% \ Cl = \frac{\text{Mass Cl}^-}{\text{Mass sample}} \times 100$$

Judge yourself

1. Why silver nitrate is not a primary standard?

2. How dichlorofluorescein acts as indicator?

3. What type of titration takes place in Fajans method? How it differs from Volhard method?

4. Could you use Fajans method to determine the exact concentration of a ~0.01 M HCl solution? Give the reason for your answer.

5. What is effect of light on silver chloride precipitates?

EXPERIMENT 18

Determination of % purity of chlorobutol

Chlorobutol is a widely used, very effective preservative in many pharmaceuticals and cosmetic products, e.g. injections, ointments, products for eyes, ears and nose, dental preparations, etc. It has antibacterial and antifungal properties. Chlorobutol is typically used at a concentration of 0.5% where it lends long-term stability to multi–ingredient formulations

Experimental overview

The determination is based on estimation of NaCl liberated from chlorobutol on boiling with NaOH.

$$CCl_3C(CH_3)_2OH + 3NaOH \longrightarrow CCl_3C(CH_3)_2OH + 3NaCl$$
Chlorobutol

$$CCl_3C(CH_3)_2OH + NaOH \longrightarrow (CH_3)_2.C(OH).COONa$$

$$3NaCl + 3AgNO_3 \longrightarrow 3NaNO_3 + 3AgCl$$

$$AgNO_3 + NH_4SCN \longrightarrow AgSCN\downarrow + NH_4NO_3$$

$$Fe^{3+} + NH_4SCN \longrightarrow Fe\,(SCN)_3$$

$$177.5 \text{ g of } C_4H_7OCl_3 = 3000 \text{ of M } AgNO_3$$

Each ml of 0.1 M $AgNO_3$ solution = 0.005917 g of $C_4H_7OCl_3$.

Reagents required

1. **0.1 M $AgNO_3$ solution:** Prepare approximately 0.1 M $AgNO_3$ by dissolving about 8.5 g of $AgNO_3$ in 500 ml of deionized water. Mix well and store in a dark glass bottle.
2. **0.1 M NH_4SCN solution:** Dissolve 7.612 g in sufficient distilled water to produce 1000 ml.
3. 10% w/v ferric ammonium sulfate solution.
4. Nitrobenzene.
5. NaOH.
6. Nitric acid.

Procedure

1. **Standardization of 0.1 M $AgNO_3$:**
   (i) Transfer approximately one gram of reagent grade NaCl from the container in the oven into a glass weighing bottle. Allow the NaCl to cool in a desiccator for 15 to 30 min.
   (ii) Dry the unknown in an oven at 100°C for 1 hr. Allow the unknown to cool to room temperature in a desiccator. Weigh accurately about 0.15–0.20 g of the dried NaCl into 250 ml Erlenmeyer flasks. Dissolve in approximately 60 ml of deionized water.
   Note: The mass of the NaCl in the solution is important, not the volume of the solution, so you can use a graduate cylinder to measure the 60 ml of water.
   (iv) Add 10 drops of the indicator solution (dichlorofluorescein) and roughly 0.1 g of dextrin (no need to weigh the dextrin) to the NaCl solution.
   (v) Rinse the buret at least 3 times with a few ml of the approximately 0.1 M $AgNO_3$ solution. Fill the buret with the 0.1 M $AgNO_3$ solution and be sure to eliminate all bubbles in the tip before continuing.

(vi) Immediately titrate the sodium chloride solution with silver nitrate until the first permanent appearance of the pink color of the indicator.

2. **Standardization of 0.1 M NH₄SCN solution:** It is deliquescent in nature, hence need standardization.To 20 ml of 0.1 M silver nitrate, add 25 ml of water, 2 ml of 2 M nitric acid and 2 ml of ferric ammonium sulfate solution and titrate with the ammonium thiocyanate solution until a reddish color is obtained. Each ml of 0.1 M silver nitrate is equivalent to 7.612 mg of NH_4SCN.

3. **Determination of chlorobutol:** Weigh accurately about 0.2 g of chlorobutol and dissolve in 5 ml of alcohol. Add to it 5 ml of sodium hydroxide solution and boil under refluxing condition. Cool, dilute with 20 ml of distilled water, add 5 ml of nitric acid, 1 ml of nitrobenzene and 50 ml of 0.1 M $AgNO_3$ solution. Shake the mixture vigorously for 1 minute, add ferric ammonium sulfate solution and titrate the excess of silver nitrate with 0.1 M NH_4SCN solution until red color. Similarly, perform a blank titration.

Observation and calculation

1. **Calculation of molarity of standard $AgNO_3$ solution:**

$$\text{Molarity} = \frac{W \text{ (g)}}{58.44 \times V \text{ (in litre)}}$$

W = Mass of NaCl in g

V = Volume of M $AgNO_3$ solution consumed

58.44 = Mol. weight of NaCl

2. **Calculation of molarity of standard NH_4SCN solution:**

$AgNO_3 = NH_4SCN$

$M_1V_1 = M_2V_2$

$$M_2 = \frac{M_1V_1}{V_2}$$

3. **Determination of chlorobutol:**

Molecular weight of chlorobutol = 177.5

Weight of the chlorobutol = W g

Vol. of 0.1 M NH_4SCN solution consumed in sample titration = V_1 ml

Vol. of 0.1 M NH_4SCN solution consumed in blank titration = V_2 ml

Vol. of 0.1 M NH_4SCN solution reacted with used $AgNO_3$ (by sample) = $V_2 - V_1 = V$ ml

From the above equation:

1 mole of NH_4SCN = 1 mole of $AgNO_3$.

V ml of 0.1 M NH_4SCN solution = V ml of 0.1 M $AgNO_3$ solution (provided molarity of both solutions is same otherwise convert the volume of NH_4SCN into volume of $AgNO_3$).

From the above equation:

$C_4H_7OCl_3 = 3NaCl = 3AgNO_3 = 3000$ ml of M $AgNO_3$

177.5 g of $C_4H_7OCl_3 = 3000$ of M

Each ml of 0.1 M $AgNO_3$ solution = 0.005917 g of $C_4H_7OCl_3$

$$\% \text{ purity of chlorobutol} = \frac{0.005917 \times V \times \text{Molarity (cal.)}}{W \times 0.1 \text{ (molarity given)}} \times 100 = \dots \%$$

Judge yourself

1. What is the use of chlorobutol?
2. What is basis of estimation of chlorobutol?
3. Why silver nitrate is not a primary standard?
4. How endpoint is detected in the above titration?
5. Why ammonium thiocyanate needs standardization?
6. Why nitrobenzene is used in this titration?
7. What are the uses of chlorobutol?
8. What is the IUPAC name for chlorobutol?

Complexometric Titrations

Introduction

Many metal ions form slightly dissociated complex ions. The formation of these can serve as the basis of accurate and convenient titrations for such metal ions. Such determinations are referred to as **complexometric** titrations. The accuracy of these titrations is high and they offer the possibility of determinations of metal ions at concentrations at the millimole level. Many cations will form complexes in solution with a variety of substances that have a pair of unshared electrons (e.g. on N, O, S atoms in the molecule) capable of satisfying the coordination number of the metal. The metal ion acts as a Lewis acid (electron pair acceptor) and the complexing agent is a Lewis base (electron pair donor). The number of molecules of the complexing agent, called the **ligand**, will depend on the coordination number of the metal and on the number of complexing groups on the ligand molecule.

Simple complexing agents such as ammonia are rarely used as titrating agents because a sharp endpoint corresponding to a stoichiometric complex is generally difficult to achieve. This is true since the stepwise formation constants are frequently close together and not very large, and a single stoichiometric complex cannot be observed. Certain ligands, that have two or more complexing groups on the molecule, however, do form well-defined complexes and can be used as titrating agents. One such reagent that is widely used is **ethylenediaminetetraacetic acid** (EDTA).

An organic agent which has two or more groups capable of complexing with a metal ion is called a chelating agent. The complex which is formed in this manner is called a **chelate**. Titration with such a chelating agent is called a **chelometric titration** which is a particular type of complexometric titration. A pair of unshared electrons capable of complexing with a metal ion is located on each of the two nitrogen atoms and each of the four carboxyl groups. Thus, there are six complexing groups in EDTA. The EDTA (represented by the symbol H_4Y), which recognizes the fact that it is a tetraprotic acid. The four hydrogens in the formula refer to the four acidic hydrogens on the four carboxyl groups. It is the unprotonated ligand Y^{4-} that is responsible for the formation of complexes with metal ions.

The present analysis is concerned with the determination of calcium ion by the use of a complexometric titration of the type that is described above. The titration is performed by adding a standard solution of EDTA to the sample containing the calcium ions. The reaction that takes place is the following.

$$Ca^{2+} + Y^{4-} \Leftrightarrow CaY^{2-}$$

Before the equivalence point, the Ca^{2+} concentration is nearly equal to the amount of unchelated (unreacted) calcium since the dissociation of the chelate is slight. At the equivalence point and beyond, pCa is determined from the dissociation of the chelate at the given pH. The equivalence point is detected through the use of an indicator which is itself a chelating agent. The specific indicator used is Eriochrome Black T. It contains three ionizable protons and we will represent it by the formula H_3In. In neutral or somewhat basic solutions, it is a doubly dissociated ion, HIn^{2-}, which is blue in color. Eriochrome Black T cannot be used as an indicator for the titration of calcium with EDTA, since it forms too weak a complex with calcium to give a sharp endpoint. Therefore, a solution containing the magnesium complex of EDTA, MgY^{2-}, is introduced into the titration mixture. Since Ca^{2+} forms a more stable complex with EDTA than magnesium, the following reaction occurs.

$$MgY^{2-} + Ca^{2+} \Leftrightarrow CaY^{2-} + Mg^{2+}$$

The magnesium that is released in this manner then reacts with the doubly ionized ion of the Eriochrome Black T. The complex that is formed between magnesium and that ion is red, hence at the start of the Ca titration the solution is red. This reaction can be written as follows:

$$Mg^{2+} + HIn^{2-} \Leftrightarrow MgIn^- + H^+$$
$$(blue) \Leftrightarrow (red)$$

The solution is then titrated with a standard solution of EDTA. At the beginning of the titration, the EDTA reacts with the remaining calcium ion that has not been complexed. After all the calcium has reacted the next portion of EDTA reacts with the magnesium complex which was formed earlier. The added EDTA competes favorably with the red magnesium-indicator complex ($MgIn^-$), to give MgY^{2-} and HIn^{2-} and thereby giving a blue color at the endpoint.

$$MgIn^- + H^+ + Y^{4-} \Leftrightarrow MgY^{2-} + HIn^{2-}$$
$$(red) \qquad \Leftrightarrow \qquad (blue)$$

EXPERIMENT 19

Determination of total hardness, permanent hardness and temporary hardness of water by EDTA titration

Experimental overview

Hardness of water is the property by virtue of which it prevents the lathering of soap. Hardness occurs due to the presence of certain salts of Ca and Mg ions in water. These react with the sodium salts of long chain fatty acids present in the soap and are precipitated out in the form of calcium and magnesium stearate, palmitate or oleates. No lather is formed until all these ions are completely removed and thus a large amount of soap is wasted.

$$2C_{17}H_{35}COONa + CaCl_2 \longrightarrow (C_{17}H_{35}COO)_2Ca + 2NaCl$$

Sodium stearate   Calcium stearate

Hardness is of two types:

1. **Temporary or carbonate hardness:** It is caused by the presence of carbonate and bicarbonate of calcium and magnesium. It can be removed by boiling the water. This is also called alkaline hardness.

$$Ca(HCO_3)_2 \longrightarrow CaCO_3 + H_2O + CO_2$$

2. **Permanent or non-carbonate hardness:** It is caused by the presence of chlorides and sulfates of calcium and magnesium which cannot be removed by boiling. This is also called non-alkaline hardness.

The hardness of water may be determined by complexometric titration. In aqueous solution, EDTA ionizes to give two Na^+ ions and a strong chelating agent.

Disodium salt of EDTA

The titration is carried out in presence of indicator, Eriochrome Black T (EBT), which is a complex organic compound.

Eriochrome Black T
(Sodium-1-(1′-hydroxy-2′-naphthylazo)-6-nitro-2-naphthol-4-sulfonate)

The indicator when added in small amount to hard water to a pH of about 10 combines with a Ca^{2+}, Mg^{2+} ions to form a weak complex of wine red color which changes to blue when an excess drop of EDTA is added.

$$\begin{vmatrix} Ca^{2+} \\ Mg^{2+} \end{vmatrix} \begin{matrix} +\ EBT \\ Blue \end{matrix} \longrightarrow \begin{vmatrix} Ca^{2+} \\ EBT \\ Mg^{2+} \end{vmatrix} \xrightarrow{\ EDTA\ } \begin{vmatrix} Ca^{2+} \\ EDTA \\ Mg^{2+} \end{vmatrix} \begin{matrix} +\ EBT \\ \\ Blue \end{matrix}$$

Wine red

Thus, the change of wine red color to distinct blue marks the endpoint of titration.

Hardness of water is expressed as $CaCO_3$ equivalent.

Reagents required

1. **Standard hard water:** Dissolve 1.0 g of pure dry $CaCO_3$ in a small amount of dilute HCl solution. Evaporate the solution to dryness on a water bath. Dissolve the residue in a distilled water and make up the volume to 1 litre.
2. **Ammonia buffer solution:** Dissolve 70 g of NH_4Cl and add 568 ml of conc. Ammonia solution and dilute with distilled water to 1 litre.
3. **Eriochrome Black T indicator (EBT):** Dissolve 0.5 g of the dye in 100 ml of rectified spirit.
4. **0.01 M EDTA solution:** Dissolve accurately weighed 3.722 g of EDTA disodium salt in distilled water and make up the volume to 1 litre

   Note: Disodium salt is available in pure form and is soluble in water.

Procedure

1. **Standardization of 0.01 M EDTA solution:** Take 25 ml of standard hard water in a conical flask. Add 10 ml of buffer solution to it followed by 2–3 drops of Eriochrome Black T indicator. Titrate the solution against standard EDTA solution from the burette until color changes from wine red to blue at the endpoint. Note the titre value (V_1 ml).
2. **Determination of total hardness:** Take 25 ml of the supplied hard water (sample) in a conical flask. Add 10 ml of buffer solution into it followed by 2–3 drops of Eriochrome Black T indicator. Titrate slowly against EDTA solution from the burette to blue color endpoint. Note the titre value (V_2 ml).
3. **Determination of permanent hardness:** Take 25 ml of supplied hard water in a 50 ml beaker and boil gently for about 10 minutes, cool and filter into a 25 ml volumetric flask and make up the volume with distilled water. Take this solution in conical flask, add 10 ml of buffer into it followed by 2–3 drops of EBT indicator. Titrate the solution slowly with EDTA to a blue colored endpoint. Note the titre value (V_3 ml).

Observation and calculation

Standardization of EDTA solution

1 ml of standard hard water = 1 mg $CaCO_3$

V_1 ml of EDTA solution = 25 ml = 25 mg of $CaCO_3$

$$1\ ml\ of\ EDTA = \frac{25}{V_1}\ mg\ of\ CaCO_3$$

Total hardness

25 ml of hard water = V_2 ml of EDTA or $= V_2 \times \dfrac{25}{V_1}$ mg of $CaCO_3$

$$1 \text{ ml of hard water} = V_2 \times \frac{25}{V_1 \times 25} \text{ mg of CaCO}_3$$

$$1000 \text{ ml of hard water} = V_2 \times \frac{25}{V_1 \times 25} 1000 \text{ mg of CaCO}_3$$

$$\text{Total hardness} = \frac{V_2}{V_1} \times 1000 \text{ ppm} = 'x' \text{ ppm}$$

Permanent hardness

$$25 \text{ ml of hard water} = V_3 \text{ ml of EDTA or}$$

$$= V_3 \times \frac{25}{V_1} \text{ mg of CaCO}_3$$

$$1000 \text{ ml of hard water} = V_3 \times \frac{25}{V_1 \times 25} \times 1000 \text{ mg of CaCO}_3$$

$$\text{Permanent hardness} = \frac{V_3}{V_1} \times 1000 \text{ ppm} = 'y' \text{ ppm}$$

Temporary hardness = Total hardness – Permanent hardness

$$= \left| \frac{V_2}{V_1} - \frac{V_3}{V_1} \right| \times 1000 \text{ ppm} = 'z' \text{ ppm}$$

Note: The hardness of water is also classified on the basis of $CaCO_3$ (ppm) as:

Classification	ppm CaCO₃
Soft	0–60
Medium hard	61–120
Hard	121–180
Very hard	>180

Judge yourself

1. What is the difference between hard and soft water?
2. What is the principle of EDTA titrations?
3. Why hardness is generally expressed as $CaCO_3$ equivalent?
4. What are disadvantages of hard water?
5. Why pH 10 is maintained in determination of hardness by EDTA titration?
6. Water softeners remove hardness by exchanging calcium and magnesium ions with another cation. Which cation you might expect to be used?
7. Draw the structure of the $CaEDTA^{2-}$ complex. Which atoms on the EDTA molecule form bonds to the calcium?
8. Why the hardness determination titration is called complexometric titration?

EXPERIMENT 20

Determination of % purity of calcium lactate

Calcium lactate is a white crystalline salt made by the action of lactic acid on calcium carbonate. In medicine, calcium lactate is most commonly used as an antacid and also to treat calcium deficiencies. Calcium lactate is added to sugar-free foods to prevent tooth decay. When added to chewing gum containing xylitol, it increases the remineralization of tooth enamel.

Experimental overview

Calcium lactate, when calculated on the dried basis, contains 97.0–101.0% of calcium lactate $(C_6H_{10}CaO_6)$.

Disodium ethylene diamine tetracetate (EDTA) solution is used as complex forming agent to form Calcium–EDTA complex in presence of ammonia–ammonium chloride buffer. Metallic indicator, Eriochrome Black T (blue color) is used which form weak complex with calcium ion (pink-purple color). On titration comparatively more stable calcium–EDTA complex is formed. At the endpoint, calcium complex formation is completed and blue color appears due to liberation of free indicator.

Calcium EDTA complex

Magnesium sulfate is added to increase the sensitivity of indicator.

Reagents required

1. **Ammonia buffer solution:** Dissolve 70 g of NH_4Cl and add 568 ml of conc. ammonia solution and dilute with distilled water to 1 litre.
2. **Eriochrome Black T indicator (EBT):** Dissolve 0.5 g of the dye in 100 ml of rectified spirit.
3. **0.05 M EDTA solution:** Dissolve accurately weighed 18.6 g of EDTA disodium salt in distilled water and make up the volume to 1 litre.
4. **0.05 M magnesium sulfate solution:** Dissolve 2.46 g $MgSO_4 \cdot 7H_2O$ in 200 ml water.

Procedure

1. **Standardization of 0.05 M EDTA solution:** Weight accurately about 0.8 g of granulated zinc, dissolve by gentle warming in 12 ml of diluted hydrochloric acid and 0.1 ml of bromine solution. Boil to remove the excess bromine, cool, add sufficient water to produce 250 ml. Pipette 20 ml in to a conical flask and nearly neutralize with 2 M sodium hydroxide. Add about 125 ml water and sufficient ammonia buffer pH 10 to dissolve the precipitate and add 5 ml in excess. Add 50 mg of mordant black II mixture and titrate with the prepared disodium edetate solution until the solution turns to green point. Each ml of 0.05M disodium edetate solution $\equiv 0.00327$ g of zinc.

Note: (a) Discard the solution after 30 days. (b) Restandardise before use. (c) Store in amber bottle with well-fitted suitable stoppers which prevent access to atmospheric carbon dioxide.

2. **Determination of calcium lactate:**
   (a) Weigh accurately about 0.3 g of calcium lactate and dissolve in 30 ml of warm water.
   (b) Add 5 ml of 0.05M magnesium sulfate solution, 10 ml of strong ammonia buffer and titrate with 0.05M disodium ethylenediamine tetraacetate, using Eriochrome Black T as indicator.
   (c) Perform the blank titration.

Observation and calculation

1. **Standardization of EDTA solution:**

$$\text{Molarity} = \frac{W \text{ (g)} \times 20}{250 \times 327 \times V \text{ (litre)}}$$

where
W = Weight of zinc in g
V = Volume of EDTA solution consumed (in litre)
327 is the molecular weight of EDTA disodium salt

2. **Determination of calcium lactate solution:**

Molecular weight of calcium lactate = 218
Weight of sample = W g
Volume of 0.05 M EDTA solution consumed in titration of sample = V_1 ml
Volume of 0.05 M EDTA solution consumed in blank titration = V_2 ml
Difference = $V_1 - V_2 = V$ ml
Each ml of 0.05 M EDTA solution = 0.01091 g of $C_6H_{10}CaO_6$

$$\% \text{ purity of calcium lactate} = \frac{0.01091 \times V \times \text{Molarity (cal)}}{W \times 0.05 \text{ (molarity given)}} \times 100 = \text{....}\%$$

Result

The percentage purity of calcium lactate = ... %.

Judge yourself

1. What is the indicator used in this titration?
2. Why Eriochrome Black T cannot be used directly as a titrant?
3. What is the color of the doubly ionized Eriochrome Black T indicator in slightly basic solution?
5. At what pH is the Ca titration carried out?
6. What are the conditional constants for Mg^{2+} and Ca^{2+} at the pH at which the titration is carried out?
7. EDTA is used in chelation therapy. Describe briefly this treatment and the principle behind.

EXPERIMENT 21

Determination of % purity of magnesium sulfate

Magnesium sulfate is commercially available as heptahydrate, monohydrate, anhydrous or dried form containing the equivalent of 2–3 waters of hydration. Magnesium sulfate occurs naturally in seawater, mineral springs and in minerals such as kieserite and epsomite. Magnesium sulfate heptahydrate is manufactured by dissolution of kieserite in water and subsequent crystallization of the heptahydrate.

Magnesium sulfate is available as brilliant colorless crystals, granular crystalline powder or white powder with a bitter salty cooling taste. Crystals effloresce in warm, dry air. It is freely soluble in water, very soluble in boiling water, and sparingly soluble in alcohol.

Magnesium sulfate is used as a nutrient, firming agent and flavor enhancer. It is also used as a fermentation aid in the processing of beer and malt beverages. It is used for immediate control of life-threatening convulsion in the treatment of toxemias of pregnancy and in the treatment of acute nephritis in children.

Experimental overview

Magnesium sulfate contains not less than 99.0% and not more than 100.0% of $MgSO_4$, calculated with reference to ignited substance.

Many metal ions react with electron pair donors to form coordination compounds or complex ions. The formation of a particular class of coordination compounds, called chelates, are especially well suited for quantitative methods. A chelate is formed when a metal ion coordinates with two (or more) donor groups of a single ligand. Tertiary amine compounds such as ethylenadiamine-tetraacetic acid (EDTA) are widely used for the formation of chelates.

Complexometric titrations with EDTA have been reported for the analysis of nearly all metal ions. Because EDTA has four acidic protons, the formation of metal ion/EDTA complexes is dependent upon the pH. For the titration of Mg^{2+}, one must buffer the solution to a pH of 10 so that complex formation will be quantitative. The reaction of Mg^{2+} with EDTA may be expressed as:

$$Mg^{2+} + H^2Y^{2-} = MgY^{-2} + 2H^+$$

The structure of EDTA and the magnesium–EDTA complex (without the hydrogen atoms) is shown here:

EDTA

Mg-EDTA complex

The endpoint of the titration is determined by the addition of Eriochrome Black T, which forms a colored chelate with Mg^{2+} and undergoes a color change when the Mg^{2+} is released to form a chelate with EDTA.

Reagents required

1. **0.05 M EDTA solution:** Dissolve accurately weighed 18.6 g of EDTA disodium salt in distilled water and make up the volume to 1 litre.
2. **Ammonia buffer solution:** Dissolve 70 g of NH_4Cl and add 568 ml of conc. ammonia solution and dilute with distilled water to 1 litre.
3. **Eriochrome Black T indicator (EBT):** Dissolve 0.5 g of the dye in 100 ml of rectified spirit.

Procedure

1. **Standardization of 0.05 M disodium EDTA solution:** The standardization is based on titration of disodium EDTA with standard $ZnCl_2$ solution prepared from known weight of granulated zinc.

$$Zn + 2HCl \longrightarrow ZnCl_2 + H_2$$

$$ZnCl_2 + C_{10}H_{14}N_2Na_2O_8 \longrightarrow C_{10}H_{14}N_2O_8Zn + 2NaCl$$

Weigh accurately about 0.8 g of granulated zinc, dissolve by gentle warming in 12 ml of diluted hydrochloric acid and 0.1 ml of bromine solution. Boil to remove the excess bromine, cool, add sufficient water to produce 250 ml. Pipette 20 ml into a conical flask and nearly neutralize with 2 M sodium hydroxide. Add about 125 ml water and sufficient ammonia buffer pH 10 to dissolve the precipitate and add 5 ml in excess. Add 50 mg of mordant black II mixture and titrate with the prepared disodium edentate solution until the solution turns to green point. Each ml of 0.05 M disodium edetate solution $\equiv$ 0.00327 g of zinc.

Note: (a) Discard the solution after 30 days. (b) Restandardise before use. (c) Store in amber bottle with well fitted suitable stoppers which prevents access to atmospheric carbon dioxide. Standardization can also be done by titration against $CaCO_3$ or ZnO using appropriate metallic indicator.

2. **Determination of magnesium sulfate:**
   (i) Accurately weigh about 0.5 g of the ignited sample, dissolve in 5 ml of hydrochloric acid TS, Dilute, dilute with water to 100 ml, and mix.
   (ii) Transfer 50 ml of this solution into a 250 ml conical flask; add 10 ml of ammonia/ Ammonium chloride buffer TS and 0.1 ml of Eriochrome Black T indicator.
   (iii) Titrate with 0.05 M disodium EDTA until the color of red-purple solution changes to blue.
   (iv) Perform a blank titration.

Observation and calculation

1. **Standardization of EDTA solution:**

$$Molarity = \frac{W \text{ (g)} \times 20}{250 \times 327 \times V \text{ (litre)}}$$

where W = Weight of zinc in g.
$\quad V$ = Volume of EDTA consumed (in litre).
$\quad$ 327 is the molecular weight of EDTA salt

2. **Determination of magnesium sulfate:**

   Molecular weight of $MgSO_4$ = 120.39

   Weight of sample = W g or 0.5 g as indicated in the procedure

   Volume of 0.05 M EDTA consumed in titration of sample = V_1 ml

   Volume of 0.05 M EDTA consumed in blank titration = V_2 ml

   Difference = $V_1 - V_2 = V$ ml

   $MgSO_4 = Mg^{2+} = C_{10}H_{14}N_2Na_2O_8$

   120.39 g $MgSO_4$ = 1000 ml of M $C_{10}H_{14}N_2Na_2O_8$ solution

   Each ml of 0.05 M EDTA solution = 0.006019 g of $MgSO_4$

   V ml of 0.05 M EDTA solution = $0.006019 \times V$ g of $MgSO_4$

   50 ml of sample solution contains $0.006019 \times V$ g of $MgSO_4$

   100 ml of sample solution contains $0.006019 \times V \times 2$ g of $MgSO_4$

   0.5 g of sample contains $0.006019 \times V \times 2$ g of $MgSO_4$

$$\% \text{ purity of magnesium sulphate} = \frac{0.006019 \times V \times \text{Molarity (cal.)}}{0.5 \times 0.05 \text{ (molarity given)}} \times 100 = ...\%$$

Result

The percentage purity of magnesium sulfate = ... %.

Judge yourself

1. What is common name for magnesium sulfate?
2. What is the use of magnesium sulfate?
3. What are the various methods to standardize EDTA solution?
4. Draw the structure of magnesium–EDTA complex.
5. How magnesium sulfate acts as cathartic?

EXPERIMENT 22

Determination of % purity of zinc sulfate

Zinc sulfate ($ZnSO_4$) is a colorless crystalline, water-soluble chemical compound. The hydrated form, $ZnSO_4 \cdot 7H_2O$, the mineral goslarite, was historically known as "white vitriol". It is used as an astringent and emetic.

Experimental overview

A complexometric titration is a titration in which substance is to be determined is a metal ion in solution. In this experiment, the metal to be determined is Zn^{2+} ion and the complexing agent is EDTA, H_4EDTA.

$$\underset{\text{HOOCCH}_2}{\overset{\text{HOOCCH}_2}{\diagdown}} NCH_2CH_2N \underset{\text{CH}_2\text{COOH}}{\overset{\text{CH}_2\text{COOH}}{\diagup}}$$

EDTA

The terminal hydrogen atoms are acidic and complete ionization results in the EDTA, $EDTA^{4-}$, the ion complexes with zinc by forming coordinate covalent bonds between Zn^{2+} and two nitrogen atoms and four oxygen atoms.

$$Zn^{2+} + EDTA^{4-} \rightleftharpoons ZnEDTA^{2-}$$

The equilibrium constant for this reaction is 3.2×10^{16}, indicating a very stable complex.

The indicator used to signal the endpoint of the titration is Eriochrome Black T. The indicator molecule is a dye that is also a complexing agent and triprotic acid, H_3In^{2-}. The color of the indicator depends on the degree of ionization, H_2In^- is red and HIn^{2-} is blue. To get an easily detectable color change, the solution is buffered at a pH of about 9.2.

For the titration, the solution containing zinc ion is first buffered, then the indicator is added. The indicator immediately forms a wine red complex with zinc ion, $ZnIn^-$. Only about 1% of the total zinc ion concentration is complexed. When the titrant is added, it first forms complex with the free zinc ion forming a colorless $ZnEDTA^{4-}$ ion. When all of the free zinc has been complexed, the $EDTA^{4-}$ will take zinc from the $ZnIn^-$ complex, the $ZnEDTA^{2-}$ complex is stronger. The wine-red of $ZnIn^-$ complex will begin to disappear and blue color of HIn^{2-} will appear.

$$\underset{\substack{\text{Wine red Colorless}}}{ZnIn^- + H_2EDTA^{2-}} \longrightarrow \underset{\substack{\text{Colorless}}}{ZnEDTA^{2-}} + \underset{\substack{\text{Blue}}}{HIn^{2-}} + H^+$$

The buffer absorbs H+ ion that is released and maintain the pH close to 9. If the solution becomes too acidic, the indicator that is released takes the form H_2In^-, which is red. The red to blue color will not be observed.

Reagent required

1. **0.05 M EDTA solution:** Dissolve accurately weighed 18.6 g of EDTA disodium salt in distilled water and make up the volume to 1 litre.
2. **Ammonia buffer solution:** Dissolve 70 g of NH_4Cl and add 568 ml of conc. ammonia solution and dilute with distilled water to 1 litre.
3. **Eriochrome Black T indicator (EBT):** Dissolve 0.5 g of the dye in 100 ml of rectified spirit.

Procedure

1. **Standardization of 0.05 M disodium EDTA solution:** The standardization is based on titration of disodium EDTA with standard $ZnCl_2$ solution prepared from known weight of granulated zinc.

$$Zn + 2HCl \longrightarrow ZnCl_2 + H_2$$

$$ZnCl_2 + C_{10}H_{14}N_2Na_2O_8 \longrightarrow C_{10}H_{14}N_2O_8Zn + 2NaCl$$

Weight accurately about 0.8 g of granulated zinc, dissolve by gentle warming in 12 ml of diluted hydrochloric acid and 0.1 ml of bromine solution. Boil to remove the excess bromine, cool, add sufficient water to produce 250 ml. Pipette 20 ml in to a conical flask and nearly neutralize with 2 M sodium hydroxide. Add about 125 ml water and sufficient ammonia buffer pH 10 to dissolve the precipitate and add 5 ml in excess. Add 50 mg of mordant black II mixture and titrate with the prepared disodium edentate solution until the solution turns to green point.

Each ml of 0.05 M disodium edetate solution $\equiv$ 0.00327 g of zinc.

Note: (a) Discard the solution after 30 days. (b) Restandardise before use. (c) Store in amber bottle with well-fitted suitable stoppers which prevent access to atmospheric carbon dioxide. Standardization can also be done by titration against $CaCO_3$ or ZnO using appropriate metallic indicator.

2. **Determination of zinc sulfate:**
   (i) Accurately weigh about 0.3 g of the ignited sample, dissolve in 100 ml of water.
   (ii) Add 5 ml of ammonia/ammonium chloride buffer TS and 0.1 ml of Eriochrome Black T indicator.
   (iii) Titrate with 0.05 M disodium EDTA until the color of red-purple solution changes to deep blue.
   (iv) Perform a blank titration.

Observation and calculation

1. **Standardization of EDTA solution:**

$$\text{Molarity} = \frac{W\,(g) \times 20}{250 \times 327 \times V\,(\text{in litre})}$$

where W = Weight of zinc in g.
$\qquad V$ = Volume of EDTA consumed in ml.

2. **Determination of zinc sulfate:**
   Weight of sample = W g
   Volume of 0.05 M EDTA consumed in titration of sample = V_1 ml
   Volume of 0.05 M EDTA consumed in blank titration = V_2 ml
   Difference = $V_1 - V_2$ = V ml
   $ZnSO_4 = Zn^{2+} = C_{10}H_{14}N_2Na_2O_8$
   Each ml of 0.05 M EDTA solution = 0.01438 g of $ZnSO_4.7H_2O$

$$\% \text{ purity of zinc sulphate} = \frac{0.01438 \times V \times \text{Molarity (cal.)}}{W \times 0.05\,(\text{molarity given})} \times 100 = ...\%$$

Result

The percentage purity of zinc sulfate = ... %.

Judge yourself

1. What is common name for zinc sulfate?
2. What is the use of zinc sulfate?
3. Ammonia forms good complex $Zn(NH_3)_4^{2+}$ with zinc ions but it is not used as titrant for its quantitative estimation. Why?

4

Redox Titrations

Introduction

Redox reactions are the most diverse of the four main classes of inorganic aqueous reactions (acid–base, precipitation, complexation and redox). In principle, redox titrations can be used to analyze for any oxidizing or reducing agent substances. However, many redox reactions are either too slow or have inconsistent stoichiometry. The stability of titrant and analyte solutions can also be a problem.

Nevertheless, a wide variety of analytes can be conveniently determined by redox titrations.

General considerations

Consider a generic redox half-reaction:

$$ox + ne^- \rightleftharpoons red$$

A chemical (i.e. ox in this equation) that pulls electrons from another substance is an oxidizing agent, while a chemical (red) that forces another substance to accept electrons is a reducing agent. Together, ox/red form a redox couple; redox couples are analogous to acid/base conjugate pairs. And just like acid–base reactions, the "conjugate" of a strong oxidizing agent is a weak reducing agent.

The strength of oxidizing/reducing agents can be deduced by the standard reduction potential: a very positive standard potential indicates a strong oxidizing agent, while a low positive or a negative potential is characteristic of a strong reducing agent.

The strength of an oxidizing or reducing agent is very often dependent on pH. There is a general rule of thumb: acidic conditions tend to make oxidizing agents more powerful and render reducing agents less reactive. Some few redox reagents are relatively insensitive to pH, which can be an advantage. Most redox reagents are stable (if they are stable at all!) only within a certain pH range.

Common titrants
Reducing agents

- Reducing agents are not stable in air (undergo air oxidation) and so are not often used. Here are a few titrants.
- The two most common reducing titrants are ferrous ammonium sulfate (FAS) and sodium thiosulfate. Procedures using these titrants are capable of determining the concentrations of analytes that are (at least) moderately strong oxidizing agents.

Ferrous ammonium sulfate (FAS or Mohr's salt), $(NH_4)_2Fe(SO_4)_2$

- The ferrous ion is a fairly weak reducing agent:

$$Fe^{2+} \longrightarrow Fe^{3+} + e^- \qquad E^\circ = 0.771 \text{ V}$$

  The use of ferrous ion as a titrant is limited to the analysis of moderately strong oxidizing agents; it is used for the direct titration of a few metals such as U(VI), Mo(VI) and V(IV). Probably the most important use of FAS is in back-titrations of dichromate and other reasonably strong oxidants.
- Solutions of FAS are most stable under acidic conditions (in 0.5 M H_2SO_4); still, the solution is stable only for about a day. Standardization is done with potassium dichromate, $K_2Cr_2O_7$.

Sodium thiosulfate, $Na_2S_2O_3$

- Thiosulfate is a moderately strong reducing agent:

$$2S_2O_3^{2-} \longrightarrow S_4O_6^{2-} + 2e^- \qquad E^\circ = 0.09 \text{ V}$$

- Thiosulfate is actually not suitable for the direct analysis of most oxidizing agents, since reactions with thiosulfate tend to produce also produce sulfite and sulfate. However, it is widely used in back-titrations of iodine that is produced by the reactions of oxidizing agents with iodide, another reducing agent (this procedure is called iodometry).
- Thiosulfate solutions are standardized with iodine which has been prepared by acidifying primary standard potassium iodate in the presence of a slight excess of potassium iodide:

Acidic solution :

$$IO_3^- + 5I^- + 6H^+ \longrightarrow 3I_2(aq) + 3H_2O$$

  The titration reaction between iodine and thiosulfate is fairly straightforward:

$$I_2 + 2S_2O_3^{2-} \longrightarrow 2I^- + S_2O_6^{2-}$$

- Alkaline solutions of sodium thiosulfate are fairly stable.

Oxidizing agents

- Used for the analysis of reducing agents. Pre-reduction of analyte is common; analyte is often unstable in reduced form, and care must be taken in sample handling.

Potassium permanganate, $KMnO_4$

- Used since the mid-1800's – one of the earliest titrimetric agents.
- A strong oxidant:

$$MnO_4^- + 4H^+ + 3e^- \longrightarrow MnO_2(s) + 2H_2O \qquad E^\circ = 1.692 \text{ V}$$

- Standardized with sodium oxalate, $Na_2C_2O_4$.
- Can be used for the analysis of many reducing agents, weak or strong. Examples are:

$$Br^-, H_2O_2, NO_2^-, Fe^{2+}, As^{3+}, Sb^{3+}, Ti^{3+}$$

Ceric sulfate, $Ce(SO_4)_2$

- Another strong oxidant, just about as strong as permanganate

$$Ce^{2+} + e^- \longrightarrow Ce^{3+} \qquad E^\circ = 1.692 \text{ V}$$

- Standardized with $Na_2C_2O_4$. Alternately, arsenic trioxide can be used.
  Titrant is very stable in acid solutions; it precipitates in alkaline solutions.
- Almost anything that can be done with potassium permanganate can be done more conveniently with ceric sulfate.

Potassium dichromate, $K_2Cr_2O_7$

- Historically important; like permanganate, used since mid–1800's.
- A moderately strong oxidizing agent; oxidizing ability depends strongly on pH, decreasing rapidly as solution becomes more neutral.

$$Cr_2O_7^{2-} + 14H + 6e^- \longrightarrow 2Cr^{3+} + 7H_2O \qquad E^o = 1.36 \text{ V}$$

- Available in sufficient purity to be its own primary standard; in fact, it is the most common reagent used to standardize reducing titrants. If necessary, dichromate solutions can be standardized with $Na_2C_2O_4$.
- Most common applications: analysis of iron content of ores.

Titrations involving iodine, I_2

General applicability

- An important class of techniques: can be used to analyze moderately strong oxidants or reductants.

  Advantage of moderate strength as a redox reagent: better selectivity.
- The standard reduction of iodine is

$$I_2(aq) + 2e^- \longrightarrow 2I^- \qquad E^o = 0.621 \text{ V}$$

- Iodine is a moderate oxidizing agent; iodide is a moderate reducing agent. There are two classes of titrations involving iodine:

  (a) *Iodimetry*, which is based on the direct reaction between the analyte and iodine. Since iodine is an oxidizing agent, iodimetry is used for the analysis of reductants. In this reaction, iodine is converted into iodide, which can be detected by using starch solution as indicator.

  (b) *Iodometry,* which is based on the reaction between the analyte and an unmeasured excess of iodide to produce iodine, which is measured by titration with thiosulfate. The amount of iodine produced by this reaction is stoichiometrically related to the amount of analyte originally present in the solution. Since iodide is an reductant, iodometry is used for the analysis of oxidants.

- Applications of iodimetry and iodometry are extensive.

  Remember: Iodimetry (analyte reacts with iodine) is for the analysis of reducing agents, while iodometry (production of iodine by reaction of analyte with iodide, followed by back-titration with thiosulfate) is for the analysis of oxidizing agents. Titrations involving iodine are more selective than those involving more powerful redox reagents.

Iodine aquatic chemistry

Iodine crystals are only sparingly soluble in water, so the standard potential listed earlier for iodine gives a misleading impression of the strength of iodine as an oxidizing agent. Usually, iodine is prepared by dissolution in a solution of concentrated potassium iodide, due to the formation of the triiodide ion:

$$I_2(aq) + I^- \rightleftharpoons I_3^-$$

This reaction allows iodine to dissolve. However, the actual concentration of I_2 (aq) remains low; thus, the oxidizing power still does not approach that of 1 M I_2 (aq). Due to the presence of triiodide, the following reaction is often used to represent iodine oxidation during a titration.

$$I_3^-(aq) + 2e^- \longrightarrow 3I^-(aq)$$

The oxidizing ability of iodine solutions is not very dependent on pH; however, in alkaline solutions (pH >8), iodine disproportionates to iodate and iodide:

$$\text{Alkaline solution: } 3I_2 + 3H_2O \rightleftharpoons IO_3^- + 5I^- + 6H^+$$

Note that this reaction is quite reversible: upon acidification, the reaction shifts to the left as iodate reacts with iodide to form iodine.

Preparation of titrant solutions

- Iodine titrant solutions are usually prepared by dissolving solid iodine in potassium iodide solutions.
  The solution may be standardized with primary standard sodium oxalate or with sodium thiosulfate that has been previously standardized.
- Sodium thiosulfate is the reducing agent that is universally used for the back-titration of iodine produced in iodometry. This titration reaction is stoichiometric and fairly rapid:

$$I_2 + 2S_2O_3^{2-} \longrightarrow 2I^- + S_4O_6^{2-}$$

- Sodium thiosulfate titrant is prepared simply by dissolving the salt in water and storing under slightly basic conditions. It is standardized with potassium iodate that has been acidified in excess iodide.

Iodine/triiodide solutions are unstable for a variety of reasons. First of all, aqueous iodine exerts a significant vapor pressure. Also, under acidic conditions iodide is slowly air-oxidized to produce iodine. Finally, under alkaline conditions, iodine will is proportionate to produce iodide and iodate, as mentioned previously. Thus, iodine solutions are generally most stable at neutral pH values. Iodine titrant solutions must be standardized fairly frequently.

Endpoint detection for redox titrations

- It is probably worthwhile to mention that starch is an excellent chemical indicator for titrations involving iodine.
- Potentiometric detection with an inert indicator electrode (e.g. Pt) is a general method for following redox titrations.
- Amperometric detection can also be used in many cases.
- Many redox titrants are colored (e.g. permanganate or iodine) and so photometric detection can also be used to follow the course of the titration.

EXPERIMENT 23

Determination of hydrogen peroxide by redox titration

Peroxy compounds, i.e. those including oxygen–oxygen bonds in covalent molecules, or O_2^{2-} ions in ionic substances, are well known and used for a variety of purposes. The simplest covalent compound containing the oxygen–oxygen bond (other than O_2) is hydrogen peroxide, H_2O_2, which in dilute aqueous solution (typically 3%) is used as a common topical antiseptic and disinfectant. Therefore, one of its common uses is to clean wounds to prevent infection. It may also be used as mouth rinse to help in removing mucus or to relieve minor mouth irritation. This product works by releasing oxygen when it is applied to the affected area. The release of oxygen causes foaming, which helps to remove dead skin and clean the area. Hydrogen peroxide in more concentrated solutions is used to bleach hair. In very concentrated solution (90%), hydrogen peroxide has been used as an oxidizer for rocket propulsion.

Hydrogen peroxide is usually encountered in the form of an aqueous solution containing about 6 per cent, 12 per cent or 30 per cent hydrogen peroxide, and frequently referred to as '20-volume', '40-volume', and '100-volume' hydrogen peroxide respectively; this terminology is based upon the volume of oxygen liberated when the solution is decomposed by boiling. Thus 1 ml of '100-volume' hydrogen peroxide will yield 100 ml of oxygen measured at standard temperature and pressure.

Experimental overview

$KMnO_4$, is a stronger oxidizing agent than H_2O_2 and reacts quantitatively with it according to the reaction:

$$2MnO_4^- + 5H_2O_2 + 6H^+ \rightarrow 2Mn^{2+} + 5O_2 + 8H_2O$$

This forms the basis of the method of analysis given below. Potassium permanganate is intensely purple, even in dilute aqueous solution. Manganous ion Mn^{+2}, is almost colorless at the same concentrations. It is therefore expected that if we add permanganate to a solution of hydrogen peroxide, the violet color will disappear as long as there is any H_2O_2 to react with the permanganate. Once the H_2O_2 is consumed, the purple color of permanganate is expected to persist. This feature makes it unnecessary to use an indicator to signal the endpoint of the reaction—the permanganate ion is the indicator. The solution will turn from clear to purple when the first drop of excess $KMnO_4$ is added to the titration container at the endpoint, slight excess of $KMnO_4$ imparts the pink color.

It is good practice to use a fairly high concentration of acid and a reasonably low rate of addition in order to reduce the danger of forming manganese dioxide, which is an active catalyst for the decomposition of hydrogen peroxide.

Reagents required

1. **0.02 M potassium permanganate ($KMnO_4$) solution:** Weigh 3.2 g of $KMnO_4$ into a 1 litre beaker. Add 500 ml of water and stir until all the $KMnO_4$ is in solution. Boil for one hour, cool, and filter through a fritted glass crucible into a 1 liter volumetric flask. Dilute to volume and mix well. Store in a dark-colored bottle.
2. Sodium oxalate ($Na_2C_2O_4$).
3. 1.0 M sulfuric acid solution. Add 30.00 ml of concentrated H_2SO_4 slowly in 970.00 ml of water. Make up the volume (to one litre) if necessary.

Procedure

1. **Standardization of 0.02 M potassium permanganate solution:** The organic matter present in potassium permanganate may cause decomposition reaction to produce MnO_2. The decomposition is enhanced in light or at high temperature. Hence, it needs standardization. Potassium permanganate solutions may be standardised using arsenic (III) oxide or sodium oxalate as primary standards.

   (i) Weigh (to the nearest 0.1 mg) about 0.15 to 0.20 g of dry sodium oxalate into a 500 ml Erlenmeyer flask. Add 200 ml of water, 50 ml of H_2SO_4, and a few glass beads.

   (ii) Heat the solution to boiling on a hot plate. Remove the flask from heat and titrate with the potassium permanganate solution until the first appearance of a faint pink color that persists for 30 seconds. Each ml of 0.02 M $KMnO_4$ = 6.7 mg of $Na_2C_2O_4$.

   The reaction between permanganate ion and oxalate ion in acidic aqueous solution is described by the following equation.

   $$2MnO_4^- + 5Na_2C_2O_4 + 6H^+ \rightarrow 2Mn^{2+} + 10CO_2 + 8H_2O$$

   Note: Do not let the temperature of the solution in the flask fall below 50°C before the endpoint is reached.

2. **Determination of hydrogen peroxide:**

   (i) Rinse a 25 ml pipet twice with about 5 ml of your hydrogen peroxide solution.

   (ii) Transfer **25.00** ml of the solution into a clean 250.0 ml volumetric flask using a 25 ml transfer pipet. Add distilled water up to the lower neck of the volumetric flask. Cap the flask and mix the solution thoroughly. When the solution is mixed, dilute with additional distill water to the mark on the volumetric flask (use a dropper if necessary). Mix again. This represents a tenfold dilution (10.00 X). 25.00 ml of the dilute solution contains only 2.500 ml of the original solution of hydrogen peroxide.

   (iii) Transfer **25.00** ml of the diluted hydrogen peroxide solution into a clean, but not necessarily dry, 125 ml Erlenmeyer flask. Add 10 ml of sulfuric acid solution using a 10 ml graduated cylinder.

   (iv) Titrate the solution with potassium permanganate. In this case, no heating of the solution is required.

   Repeat above procedure twice more. If the volumes of $KMnO_4$ you use in these titrations have a percent deviation larger than 2%, repeat the titration. Note that each titration is performed on the same volume of hydrogen peroxide solution.

   Therefore, if the concentration of the hydrogen peroxide solution is uniform and the pipet has been used properly, the volume of potassium permanganate required should be the same in each titration.

Observation and calculation

1. **Standardization of 0.02 M KMNO$_4$ solution:**

   Sample calculation:

   Molecular weight of $Na_2C_2O_4$ = 134

   Volume of $KMnO_4$ solution consumed: 20.0 ml

   Step 1: Write the equation:

   $$2MnO_4^- + 5C_2O_4^{2-} + 16H^+ \longrightarrow 2Mn^{-2} + 10CO_2 + 8H_2O$$

Step 2: Work out moles ratio:

$$2 \text{ moles of } MnO_4^- = 5 \text{ moles of } C_2O_4^{2-}$$

$$\text{Molarity of } KMnO_4 \text{ solution} = \frac{\text{Weight of sodium oxalate (g)} \times 0.4}{134 \times \text{Volume of } KMnO_4 \text{ solution (L)}}$$

$$= \frac{0.15 \times 0.4}{134 \times 0.020}$$

The factor 0.4 is required because 5 moles of oxalate react with 2 moles of MnO_4^- (1 mole = 0.4 mole) = 0.022 M.

2. **Determination of H_2O_2:**

V = ml of potassium permanganate used in titration
M = Molarity of potassium permanganate
W = ml of sample into flask
1 ml of 0.1 N $KMnO_4$ solution = 0.001701 g of H_2O_2
Dilution factor = 10

The amount of H_2O_2 (w/v) in 2.5 ml H_2O_2 solution (undiluted) or 25 ml of diluted H_2O_2 solution

$$= \frac{(V) \,(\text{Molarity cal.}) \,(0.001701)}{0.02 \,(\text{molarity given})}$$

The amount of H_2O_2 (w/v) in 25 ml H_2O_2 solution (undiluted)

$$= \frac{(V) \,(\text{Molarity cal.}) \,(0.001701)(10)}{0.02 \,(\text{molarity given})}$$

$$\% \text{ of } H_2O_2 \,(w/v) = \frac{(V) \,(\text{Molarity cal.}) \,(0.001701)(10)}{0.02 \times 25} \times 100$$

Result

The % of H_2O_2 (w/v) is = ... w/v.

Note: If the proper equipment is available, this titration can be done potentiometrically.

Judge yourself

1. In the reaction of $KMnO_4$ (aq) with H_2O_2 (aq), which species is oxidized and which is reduced? Explain.
2. Why sulfuric acid is added in permanganate titration?
3. What is self indicator? Name the other titrant that acts as self indicator.
4. In the potassium permanganate titration, sulfuric acid is used to determine the concentration of permanganate. Why hydrochloric acid or nitric acid cannot be used instead of sulfuric acid?
5. Why sodium oxalate solution is warmed to 50°C temperature in standardisation of $KMnO_4$ solution?

EXPERIMENT 24

Determination of ferrous sulfate by redox titration

Ferrous sulfate occurs as crystal (heptahydrate) called ferrous sulfate (crystal) and a dried substance (monohydrate) called ferrous sulfate (dry). Ferrous sulfate is used to treat iron deficiency anemia (a lack of red blood cells caused by having too little iron in the body).

Experimental overview

Ferrous sulfate (crystals) contains 98.0–104% of ferrous sulfate heptahydrate ($FeSO_4.7H_2O = 278.02$) and ferrous sulfate (dry) contains not less than 85.0% ferrous sulfate ($FeSO_4 = 151.91$).

Ferrous sulfate (reducing agent) is determined by redox titration with standard $KMnO_4$ (oxidizing agent) according to following reaction.

$$2KMnO_4 + 8H_2SO_4 + 10FeSO_4 \longrightarrow 2MnSO_4 + 5Fe_2 (SO_4)_3 + K_2SO_4 + 8H_2O$$

Ferrous sulfate is oxidized into ferric sulfate. At the endpoint, a slight excess of $KMnO_4$ imparts pink color.

Reagents required

1. 0.02 M potassium permanganate solution. Weigh 3.2 g of $KMnO_4$ into a 1 litre beaker. Add 500 ml of water and stir until all the $KMnO_4$ is in solution. Boil for one hour, cool, and filter through a fritted glass crucible into a 1 liter volumetric flask. Dilute to volume and mix well. Store in a dark colored bottle.
2. Sodium oxalate ($Na_2C_2O_4$).
3. 1.0 M sulfuric acid solution. Add 30.00 ml of concentrated H_2SO_4 slowly in 970.00 ml of water. Make up the volume to 1 litre.

Procedure

1. **Standardization of 0.02 M potassium permanganate solution:**
   (i) Weigh (to the nearest 0.1 mg) about 0.3 g of dry sodium oxalate into a 500 ml Erlenmeyer flask. Add 200 ml of water, 50 ml of H_2SO_4, and a few glass beads.
   (ii) Heat the solution to boiling on a hot plate. Remove the flask from heat and titrate with the potassium permanganate solution until the first appearance of a faint pink color that persists for 30 seconds. Do not let the temperature of the solution in the flask fall below 50°C before the endpoint is reached.
2. **Determination of ferrous sulfate (powder):**
   (i) Weigh accurately about 0.5 g of ferrous sulfate, dissolve in a mixture of 25 ml of dilute sulfuric acid and 25 ml of freshly boiled and cooled distilled water.
   (ii) Titrate with 0.02 M $KMnO_4$ solution till pink color persists for 30 second.

Observation and calculation

1. **Standardization of 0.02M potassium permanganate solution:** The reaction between permanganate ion and oxalate ion in acidic aqueous solution is described by the following equation.

$$2MnO_4^- + 5C_2O_4^{2-} + 16H^+ \longrightarrow 2Mn^{-2} + 10CO_2 + 8H_2O$$

Sample calculation:

Molecular weight of $Na_2C_2O_4 = 134$

Weight of $Na_2C_2O_4 = 0.1974$ g (= 197.4 mg)

Volume of $KMnO_4$ solution = 31.34 ml

M moles of $Na_2C_2O_4$ (weight (mg)/134.00) [= 197.4/134.0] = 1.473 m moles

From the above equation:

2 mole of $KMnO_4 = 5Na_2C_2O_4$

Hence, 1 mole of $Na_2C_2O_4 = 2/5$ $KMnO_4$

1.473 M moles of $Na_2C_2O_4 = 2 \times 1.473/5 = 0.5892$ m moles $KMnO_4$

Molarity of $KMnO_4$ (mmol $KMnO_4$/ml $KMnO_4$) [= 0.5892/31.34] = 0.01880 M

Alternate method:

$$\text{Molarity of } KMnO_4 \text{ solution} = \frac{\text{Weight of sodium oxalate (g)} \times 0.4}{134 \times \text{Volume of } KMnO_4 \text{ solution (L)}}$$

$$= \frac{0.1974 \times 0.4}{134 \times 0.03134}$$

$$= 0.0188 \text{ M}$$

2. **Determination of ferrous sulfate:**

Weight of sample = W g

From the above equation:

$$2 \text{ moles of } KMnO_4 = 10FeSO_4.7H_2O$$

1000 ml of 1 M $KMnO_4$ solution = $1KMnO_4$ or $5FeSO_4.7H_2O$

1000 ml of 0.02 KMnO4 solution = 5×0.02 $FeSO_4.7H_2O$

$$= 1/10 \text{ } FeSO_4.7H_2O \text{ or } 27.8 \text{ g of } FeSO_4.7H_2O$$

$$V \text{ ml of 0.02 } KMnO_4 \text{ solution} = \frac{27.8}{1000} \times V \text{ g of } FeSO_4.7H_2O$$

$$\% \text{ purity of ferrous sulfate} = \frac{0.0278(V) \text{ (Molarity cal)}}{W(0.02)} \times 100 = ... \% \text{ of } FeSO_4.7H_2O$$

Judge yourself

1. What is green vitrol?
2. What is need of standardization of $KMnO_4$ solution?
3. Why the molar solution of $KMnO_4$ is preferred for quantitative estimation?
4. How potassium permanganate solution is filtered?
5. Mention the various primary standards useful for standardization of potassium permanganate solution.

EXPERIMENT 25

Determination of ferrous sulfate content in tablets

Experimental overview

Ferrous sulfate (reducing agent) is titrated with ceric sulfate (oxidizing agent). Ferrous sulfate is oxidized into ferric sulfate.

$$2FeSO_4 + Ce(SO_4)_2 \longrightarrow Fe(SO_4)_3 + Ce_3(SO_4)_3$$

At the endpoint, ferroin sulfate (complex) (indicator, red color) is oxidized into ferric form which is blue in color.

$$Fe(C_{12}H_8N_2)^{2+} \longrightarrow Fe(C_{12}H_8N_2)^{3+} + e$$

Ferrous complex   Ferric complex
(red)   (blue)

Reagents required

1. **0.1 M ceric ammonium sulfate solution:** Dissolve 63.26 g of cerium ammonium sulfate in a mixture of 500 ml of water and 30 ml of sulfuric acid. Allow to cool and dilute to 1000.0 ml with water.
2. Ferroin sulfate.
3. Sulfuric acid.
4. Arsenic trioxide.

Procedure

1. **Standardization of 0.1 M ceric ammonium sulfate solution:** The standardization is based upon the oxidation of sodium arsenite by the cerric component of the salt, using ferroin as indicator.

$$NaAsO_2 + 2H_2O \longrightarrow NaH_2AsO_4 + 2H^+ + 4e$$

$$4[Ce^{4+} + e \longrightarrow Ce^{3+}]$$

Sodium arsenite is formed by dissolving the arsenic trioxide in NaOH solution.
Accurately weigh about 0.2 g of arsenic trioxide and dissolve by gently heating in 15 ml of 0.2 M sodium hydroxide. Add to the clear solution 50 ml of sulfuric acid (~100 g/L) TS, 0.15 ml of a 2.5 mg/ml solution of osmium tetraoxide in sulfuric acid (~100 g/L), and 0.1 ml of ferroin sulfate indicator. Titrate the solution with the cerric ammonium sulfate solution until the red color disappears. Titrate slowly as the endpoint is approached. Osmium tetraoxide acts as a catalyst.

2. **Determination of ferrous sulfate in tablet:**
   (i) Weigh accurately 20 tablets and find out the average weight.
   (ii) Powder the tablets and accurately weigh the powder equivalent to 0.5 g of ferrous sulfate.
   (iii) Dissolve in a mixture of 25 ml of dilute sulfuric acid and 25 ml of freshly boiled and cooled distilled water. Add few drops of ferroin sulfate indicator.
   (iv) Titrate with 0.1 M cerric ammonium sulfate solution till blue color persists for 30 second.
   (v) Similarly, perform the blank titration.

Observation and calculation

1. **Standardization of 0.1 M cerric ammonium sulfate solution:**

   Sample calculation:

   Molecular weight of arsenic trioxide = 197.84

   Weight of arsenic trioxide = 0.1984 g (= 198.4 mg)

   Volume of cerric ammonium sulfate solution consumed = 30.00 ml

   M moles of As_2O_3 = (weight (mg)/197.84 [= 198.4/197.84] = 1.002 m moles

   From the above equation:

   4 mole of Ce^{4+} = 1 mole of $NaASO_2$

   Hence, 1 mole of $NaAsO_2$ (or As_2O_3) = 4 Ce^{4+}

   1.002 M moles of $NaAsO_2$ (or As_2O_3) = 4 × 1.002 = 4.008 m moles Ce^{4+}

   Molarity of Ce^{4+} = (mmol Ce^{4+}/ml cerric ammonium sulfate [= 4.008/30] = 0.133 M

   Alternatively, molarity of cerric ammonium sulfate solution

   $$= \frac{\text{Weight of } As_2O_3 \text{ (in g)}}{197.84 \times \text{Volume (in L)}}$$

   $$= \frac{0.1984 \times 4}{197.84 \times 0.030}$$

   $$= 0.133 \text{ M}$$

2. **Determination of ferrous sulfate in tablet:**

   Molecular weight of ferrous sulfate = 278

   Average weight of tablet = W_1

   Weight of powder equivalent to 0.5 g of ferrous sulfate = W_2 g

   Volume of 0.1 M cerric ammonium sulfate solution consumed (in sample) = V_1 ml

   Volume of 0.1 M cerric ammonium sulfate solution consumed (in blank) = V_2 ml

   The difference between sample and blank titration = $V_1 - V_2 = V$ ml

   From the above equation:

   1 mole cerric ammonium sulfate = 1 mole of $FeSO_4.7H_2O$

   1000 ml of 0.1 M cerric sulfate = $0.1FeSO_4.7H_2O$

   V ml of 0.1 M cerric sulfate solution = $0.0278(V)$ g of $FeSO_4.7H_2O$

   The content of ferrous sulfate per average weight tablet = $\dfrac{0.0278(V) \text{ molarity (cal)}}{W_2 \times \text{molarity (given)}} \times W_1$

   $$\% \text{ content} = \frac{\text{Practical value}}{\text{Theoretical value}} \times 100$$

Judge yourself

1. Why sulfuric acid is added in ceric sulfate titration?
2. What is ferroin? Mention its structure.
3. Why ferrous sulfate tablet is generally not titrated with $KMnO_4$ solution?
4. What are various other primary standards to standardize ceric sulfate?

EXPERIMENT 26

Determination of metamizole content in analgin tablets

Metamizole sodium is a non-steroidal anti-inflammatory drug (NSAID), commonly used in many countries as a powerful painkiller and fever reducer. It is better known under the names Dipyrone, Analgin, Novalgin, and Melubrin.

Experimental overview

The determination of metamizole sodium depends upon the oxidation of the enolic group present in metamizole with iodine.

Metamizole (keto form)   Metamizole (enolic form)

Reagents required

1. Alcohol
2. **Standard 0.1 N iodine solution:** Dissolve 12.7 g of reagent grade iodine (I_2) in a solution of 40 g of potassium iodide in 25 ml of purified water. Transfer to a 1 L volumetric flask, dilute to volume with purified water and mix.
   Iodine is practically insoluble in water. It dissolves in solution of potassium iodide due to polyiodide formation, KI_3, which behaves in solution as free iodine.
3. HCl solution
4. Arsenic trioxide
5. Starch mucilage indicator

Procedure

1. **Standardization of standard iodine solution:**
A. **Procedure A:**
   (i) Dissolve accurately weighed 0.2 g of As_2O_3 in 20 ml of 1.0 N NaOH solution by warming if necessary. Add 40 ml of water, add 2 drops of methyl orange and add sufficient quantity of dilute HCl solution until yellow color changes to pink.
   As_2O_3 (primary standard) is insoluble in water but solubilized in NaOH due to formation of sodium arsenite

$$As_2O_3 + 6NaOH \longrightarrow 2Na_3AsO_3 + 3H_2O$$
$$\text{Sodium arsenite}$$

The excess of sodium hydroxide is neutralized by adding dilute HCl using methyl orange as indicator otherwise hypoiodite, NaIO or similar compound forms.

$$2NaOH + I_2 \longrightarrow NaIO + NaI + H_2O$$
$$\text{Sodium hypoiodite}$$

(ii) Then, add 2 g of sodium bicarbonate (2 g), 50 ml of water, add starch mucilage indicator and titrate with 0.1 N iodine solution until permanent blue color is produced.
Iodine oxidizes arsenite into arsenate.

$$H_3AsO_3 + H_2O + I_2 \longrightarrow H_3AsO_4 + 2HI$$

Due to strong reducing properties of HI, the oxidation with iodine is a reversible reaction. The reaction proceeds to the right by removal of hydroiodic acid by reaction with $NaHCO_3$. Sodium hydroxide or sodium carbonate cannot be used due to their reactivity with iodine. Sodium bicarbonate does not react with iodine but if an excess of iodine is added, it may react slightly.
The overall reaction is:

$$Na_3AsO_3 + I_2 + 2NaHCO_3 \longrightarrow Na_3AsO_4 + NaI + 2CO_2 + H_2O$$
$$\text{Sodium arsenite} \qquad\qquad\qquad \text{Sodium arsenate}$$

B. **Procedure B:** Using standardized 0.1 N sodium thiosulfate
   (i) Pipet (wipe the pipet before leveling) 20.0 ml of freshly standardized 0.1 N sodium thiosulfate into a 250 ml conical flask containing 50 ml of distilled water.
  (ii) Add 2 ml of starch indicator from a tip-up pipet.
 (iii) Using a 25 ml burette, titrate with the iodine being standardized. The endpoint is indicated by the appearance of the first blue color. Record the volume of iodine used for the titration.
 (iv) Repeat the standardization two more times.
  (v) Calculate the average of the three standardizations.

2. **Determination of metamizole:**
   (i) Weigh accurately 20 tablets and find out the average weight of tablet. Powder them.
  (ii) Weigh accurately powder equivalent to 0.5 g of metamizole, dissolve in a mixture of 40 ml of alcohol and 10 ml of 0.01 N HCl solution and make up the volume to 100 ml in volumetric flask.
 (iii) Shake well and filter if necessary.
 (iv) Titrate 25 ml of the filtrate with 0.1 N iodine solution till a yellow color that remains stable for 30 seconds.

Observation and calculation

1. **Standardization of 0.1 N iodine solution:**
Procedure A: Using As_2O_3
Normality of iodine is calculated as follows:

$$N = \frac{\text{Weight of } As_2O_3}{\text{ml of iodine consumed} \times 0.04946}$$

where 0.04946 is the milliequivalent weight of As_2O_3

Procedure B: Using sodium thiosulfate

$$N \text{ iodine} = \frac{(N \text{ Na}_2\text{S}_2\text{O}_3 \times \text{ml Na}_2\text{S}_2\text{O}_3)}{\text{ml iodine titrated}} = \frac{(N \text{ Na}_2\text{S}_2\text{O}_3)(20)}{\text{ml iodine}}$$

2. **Determination of metamizole:**

   Molecular weight of metamizole = 333.40

   Volume of 0.1 N iodine solution consumed by **25 ml** metamizole solution = V ml

   Average weight of tablet = W_1 g

   Weight of powder equivalent to 0.5 g of metamizole = W_2 g

   $C_{13}H_{16}N_3NaO_4S$ (metamizole) = I_2 = $2e$

   333.40 g of $C_{13}H_{16}N_3NaO_4S$ = 2000 ml of 1 N iodine solution

   166.70 g of $C_{13}H_{16}N_3NaO_4S$ = 1000 ml of 1 N iodine solution

   0.01667 g of $C_{13}H_{16}N_3NaO_4S$ = 1 ml of 0.1 N iodine solution

   V ml of 0.1 N iodine solution = $V \times 0.01667$ g of $C_{13}H_{16}N_3NaO_4S$

   100 ml or W_2 g metiamazole contain $V \times 0.01667 \times 4$ g of $C_{13}H_{16}N_3NaO_4S$

   Content of metamizole in average weight tablet

   $$= \frac{V \times 0.01667 \times 4}{W_2} \times W_1 \text{ g of } C_{13}H_{16}N_3NaO_4S$$

   $$\% \text{ of metamizole} = \frac{\text{Practical value}}{\text{Theoretical value}} \times 100$$

Judge yourself

1. What is the basis of titration?
2. Why iodine is not a primary standard?
3. How the endpoint is detected in the titration of analgin with iodine?
4. What is the mechanism of action of analgin?

EXPERIMENT 27

Determination of isoniazid by redox titration

Isoniazid is a chemotherapeutic agent that is used to kill the bacteria that cause tuberculosis (TB). Its exact mechanism of action is unknown but it is thought to prevent the bacteria from making components called mycolic acids which are needed to form cell walls. It also seems to combine with an enzyme which interferes with the cell metabolism of the bacteria. As a result of the disruption in its metabolism and without a cell wall the bacteria die.

Experimental overview

It is an example of redox titration. Isoniazid can be directly titrated using potassium bromate in strong acid condition. Potassium bromate oxidizes isoniazid into isonicotinic acid.

Isoniazid   Isonicotinic acid

Excessive BrO_3^- reacts with Br^- to form Br_2 that change the methyl red indicator into colorless form to indicate the end of the titration.

Reagents required

1. **0.01667 M potassium bromate solution:** Dissolve 2.784 g of potassium bromate in sufficient water to produce 1000 ml.
2. Potassium bromide solution.
3. Methyl red indicator.

Procedure

Determination of isoniazid in powder

  (i) Accurately weigh 0.2 g of the sample and transfer to 100 ml volumetric flask.
 (ii) Dissolve in distilled water and dilute to volume with water, mix well.
(iii) Accurately transfer 25 ml of the solution, add 0.2 g of KBr, 20 ml of dilute HCl solution and 25 ml of water and then add 1 drop of methyl red indicator.
(iv) Slowly titrate with 0.01667 M potassium bromate till the disappearance of red color.

Determination of isoniazid in tablets

  (i) Accurately weigh 20 tablets and find out the average weight of tablet. Powder finely.
 (ii) Accurately weigh a proper quantity (equivalent to about 0.2 g isoniazid) and transfer to 100 ml volumetric flask.
(iii) Dissolve with water, mix, dilute with water to volume.
(iv) Filter with dry paper, accurately transfer 25 ml of consequent filtrate, and proceed as directed in "The assay of isoniazid" with "add 0.2 g of KBr ...".

Observation and calculation

For isoniazid powder

Mol. wt. of isoniazid = 137

Weight of powder = W g of isoniazid

Molarity of potassium bromate = M

Volume of 0.01667 M $KBrO_3$ consumed = V ml

From the equation:

3 moles of isoniazid = $2KBrO_3$

Each ml of the 0.01667 M potassium bromate = 0.003429 g of $C_6H_7N_3O$

$$V \text{ ml of } 0.01667 \text{ m } KBrO_3 \text{ solution} = \frac{0.003429 \times V \times M}{0.01667} \text{ g of } C_6H_7N_3O$$

$$\text{Content of isoniazid in 100 ml solution or } W \text{ g of powder} = \frac{0.003429 \times V \times M \times 4}{0.01667} \text{ g}$$

$$\% \text{ purity} = \frac{0.003429 \times V \times M \times 4}{0.01667 \times W} \times 100$$

For isoniazid tablet:

Average weight of tablet = W_1 g

Weight of tablet powder = W_2 g

Molarity of potassium bromate = M

$$V \text{ ml of } 0.01667 \text{ m } KBrO_3 \text{ solution} = \frac{0.003429 \times V \times M}{0.01667} \text{ g of } C_6H_7N_3O$$

$$\text{Content of isoniazid in 100 ml solution or } W_2 \text{ g of powder} = \frac{0.003429 \times V \times M \times 4}{0.01667} \text{ g}$$

$$\text{Content of isoniazid in average weight tablet} = \frac{0.003429 \times V \times M \times 4}{0.01667 \times W_1} \text{ g}$$

Judge yourself

1. What is the reaction between isoniazid and potassium bromate?
2. How endpoint is detected in this titration?
3. How isoniazid acts as antituberculotic drug?
4. Name the other methods of assay of isoniazid.

EXPERIMENT 28

Determination of % purity of benzyl penicillin

Penicillin (sometimes abbreviated PCN) is a group of beta-lactam antibiotics used in the treatment of bacterial infections caused by susceptible, usually gram-positive, organisms. The sodium or potassium salt of benzyl penicillin is colorless or white powder, soluble in water.

Experimental overview

The intact penicillin molecule does not consume iodine while its hydrolytic product, penicilloic acid consumes molecule. The hydrolysis of benzyl penicillin is done by either with alkali or enzyme, lactamase. Hence, intact benzyl penicillin is allowed to react with standard iodine solution. In the same way, the benzyl penicillin after hydrolysis in presence of alkali solution is allowed to react with standard iodine solution. The difference in iodine consumption is analysed for the assay of benzyl penicillin. The method depends upon the reduction of iodine by the hydrolyzed substrate. Determined experimentally, 1 mol of hydrolyzed penicillins consumed 3.4 to 4.0 mol of iodine (I_2).

Benzyl penicillin   Penicilloic acid

Reagents required

1. **0.02 N iodine solution:** Dissolve 1.5 g of reagent grade iodine (I_2) in a solution of 8 g of potassium iodide in 25 ml of purified water. Transfer to a 1 L volumetric flask, dilute to volume with purified water and mix.

   Iodine is practically insoluble in water. It dissolves in solution of potassium iodide due to polyiodide formation, KI_3, which behaves in solution as free iodine.

2. **0.02 N sodium thiosulfate solution:** Although sodium thiosulfate ($Na_2S_2O_3 \cdot 5H_2O$, MW = 248.17) can be obtained in high purity, solutions may exhibit some decomposition reactions. Therefore, it is prudent to prepare solutions approximately, and then standardize them with a primary standard reagent.

   Boil 1 litre of distilled H_2O for several minutes, and then cool. Add about 5 g of $Na_2S_2O_3 \cdot 5H_2O$ and 0.1 g of Na_2CO_3. Stir until all crystals are dissolved and transfer to a clean bottle.

3. **Starch mucilage indicator:** Rub 1 g of soluble starch and 15 ml of H_2O into a paste. Dilute to about 500 ml with H_2O. Heat until the mixture is clear. Cool. Prepare fresh starch solution for each day of lab.

4. Potassium iodate.

Procedure

1. **Standardization of 0.02 N iodine solution:**
   (i) Pipet 25.00 ml iodine (I_2) solution into 250 ml flasks.

(ii) Add 2.00 g of potassium iodide (KI). Swirl the flask to mix thoroughly.

(iii) Add 2.0 ml 6 M HCl.

(iv) Titrate immediately with $Na_2S_2O_3$ until solution color changes from deep red to pale yellow. Add 5 ml of starch indicator (solution color goes from pale yellow to deep blue).

(v) Continue the titration till the disappearance of blue color. Note the titre value.

2. **Standardization of 0.02 N sodium thiosulfate solution:**

(i) Prepare a 0.02 N KIO_3 solution, add of potassium iodate [$KIO_3(s)$] to 100.0 ml of H_2O.

(ii) Transfer 25 ml of potassium iodate solution in conical flask.

(iii) Add 2.00 g ($\pm$ 0.01 g) potassium iodide (KI).

(iv) Add 20.0 ml of H_2O and 2 ml of 6 M HCl.

(v) Titrate immediately with $Na_2S_2O_3$ (solution color goes from deep rust to pale yellow).

(vi) Add 1 ml of starch indicator (solution color goes from pale yellow to deep blue).

(vii) Titrate till the disappearance of the blue color. Note the titre value.

3. **Determination of benzylpenicillin:**

(i) Weigh accurately about 60 mg of benzyl penicillin and dissolve in sufficient water to produce 50 ml in volumetric flask.

(ii) Transfer 10 ml of the solution to a stoppered flask, add 5 ml of 1 N NaOH solution and heat in a water-bath for 30 minutes.

(iii) Add 5.5 ml of 1 N HCl solution and 30 ml of 0.02 N iodine solution, close the flask with a wet stopper, heat in a water-bath for 30 minutes.

(iv) Titrate the excess of iodine with 0.02 N sodium thiosulfate, using starch mucilage added toward the end of titration, as indicator.

(v) To a further 10 ml of solution of benzyl penicillin prepared in the beginning add 30 ml of 0.02 N iodine, and titrate immediately with 0.02 N sodium thiosulfate, using starch mucilage added toward the end of titration, as indicator.

(vi) The difference between the two titrations represents the amount of iodine that is equivalent to the penicillin present.

Observation and calculation

1. **Standardization of 0.02 N sodium thiosulfate solution:**

Weight of potassium iodate = W g

Molecular weight of potassium iodate = 214

Equivalent weight of potassium iodate = 214/6

Normality of potassium iodate = N_2

Normality of sodium thiosulfate = (N_1) ?

Volume of sodium thiosulfate consumed = V_1 ml

Volume of potassium iodate solution = 25 ml

$$N_1 = \frac{N_2 \times 25}{V_1}$$

2. **Standardization of 0.02 N iodine solution:**

Normality of sodium thiosulfate = (N_1)

Volume of sodium thiosulfate consumed = V_1 ml

Volume of iodine solution = 25 ml

Normality of iodine solution (N_2) = ?

$$N_2 = \frac{N_1 \times V_1}{25}$$

3. **Determination of benzylpenicillin:**

   Weight of powder = W g

   Amount of 0.02 N sodium thiosulfate consumed in blank titration = V_3 ml

   Amount of 0.02 N sodium thiosulfate consumed in sample titration = V_4 ml

   Difference between two titrations = $V_3 - V_4 = V$ ml

   Each ml of 0.02 N iodine = 0.000764 gm of total penicillins, calculated as $C_{16}H_{17}O_4N_2SNa$ or to 0.000798 gm of total penicillins calculated as $C_{16}H_{17}O_4N_2SK$.

   Note: Repeat the assay using the standard preparation of penicillin to determine the exact equivalent ml of 0.02 N iodine and from this calculate the result of assay.

   V ml of 0.02 N iodine solution: 0.000764 × V g of $C_{16}H_{17}O_4N_2SNa$

   W g of sample powder = 0.000764 × V × 5 g of $C_{16}H_{17}O_4N_2SNa$

   Note: W g is dissolved in 50 ml.

   $$\% \text{ purity} = \frac{0.000764 \times V \times 5 \times N_2}{W \times 0.02} \times 100 \text{ g of } C_{16}H_{17}O_4N_2SNa$$

Judge yourself

1. What is principle involved in the estimation of benzylpenicillin?
2. Why NaOH is added in this titration?
3. Why sodium carbonate is added in the preparation of standard sodium thiosulfate solution?
4. What are various hydrolytic products in the acidic media?

EXPERIMENT 29

Determination of copper sulfate

Copper (II) sulfate is the chemical compound with the formula $CuSO_4$. The anhydrous form is a pale green or gray-white powder, whereas the pentahydrate, the most commonly encountered salt, is bright blue. This hydrated copper sulfate occurs in nature as the mineral called chalcanthite.

Copper sulfate is a very versatile chemical with extensive range of uses in industry. It is used as raw material for the production of many copper salts. Copper sulfate is generally used as insecticide in agriculture and wood industry.

Experimental overview

It contains not less than 98.5% and not more than the equivalent of 101% w/w of $CuSO_4.5H_2O$.

Copper sulfate is assayed by iodometric method. Reducing agent, KI, is added in presence of acetic acid to form cupric iodide. Acetic acid is added to form a weakly acidic solution.

Cupric iodide is unstable and decomposes into cuprous iodide and iodine. The liberated iodine is titrated with sodium thiosulfate till the solution becomes yellow. Most of the liberated iodine is reacted with sodium thiosulfate, little amount is left (indicated by yellow colour).

Starch mucilage is added towards the end because it forms stable complex with excess of iodine.

$$2CuSO_4 + 4KI \longrightarrow 2CuI_2 + 2K_2SO_4$$

$$\underset{\text{Cupric iodide}}{2CuI_2} \qquad \underset{\text{Cuprous iodide}}{Cu_2I_2 + I_2}$$

$$\underset{\substack{\text{Sodium}\\\text{thiosulfate}}}{I_2 + 2Na_2S_2O_3} \longrightarrow \underset{\substack{\text{Sodium}\\\text{tetrathionate}}}{2Na_2S_4O_6 + 2NaI}$$

The decomposition of cupric iodide into cuprous iodide and iodine is reversible, hence to make quantitative, potassium thiocyanate is added which reacts with the reaction product, cuprous iodide, to form cuprous thiocyanate. Potassium thiocyanate is added toward the end of the titration to avoid errors due to adsorption of iodine by cuprous thiocyanate.

$$Cu_2I_2 + KCNS \longrightarrow \underset{\text{Cuprous thiocyanate}}{CuCNS\downarrow + 2KI}$$

Reagents required

1. **0.1 N sodium thiosulfate:** Dissolve 25 g of sodium thiosulfate pentahydrate ($Na_2S_2O_3 \cdot 5H_2O$ and 0.1 g of sodium carbonate 800 ml of water and mix thoroughly by shaking for approximately 15 minutes. Make up the volume to 1 litre Store in a glass-stoppered reagent.
2. Potassium iodide.
3. **0.1 N potassium iodate solution:** Weigh (to the nearest 0.1 mg) about 3.57 g of dried primary standard potassium iodate (KIO_3) and transfer to a 1 liter volumetric flask. Add 400 ml of H_2O. Shake until dissolution is complete. Dilute to volume and mix well.
4. Potassium thiocyanate.
5. Acetic acid.
6. Starch mucilage.

Procedure

1. **Standardization of 0.1 N sodium thiosulfate solution:** Pipette 20.0 ml of 0.1 N potassium iodate solution into a 250 ml iodine flask containing 50 ml of H_2O. Add about 20 ml of potassium iodide (10%) and mix well. Add 25 ml of hydrochloric acid, stopper the flask, and wait five minutes. Using a 50 ml burette, titrate with the sodium thiosulfate solution until the brown triiodide color is nearly dispersed to a pale straw color. Add about 1 ml of the starch solution and titrate until the solution changes sharply from blue to colorless. Record the titration volume and calculate the normality of the sodium thiosulfate solution as shown below.

2. **Determination of copper sulfate:** Weigh accurately about 1 g of copper sulphate, dissolve in 50 ml of water, add 3 g of potassium iodide and 5 ml of acetic acid to it and titrate the liberated iodine with 0.1 N sodium thiosulfate till solution becomes light yellow in color. At this stage, add starch mucilage and 2 g of potassium thiocyanate and continue the titration until blue color disappears.

Observation and calculation

A. **Standardization of sodium thiosulfate:**

Normality of potassium iodate $= N_1$

Volume of potassium iodate solution $= 20$ ml

Normality of sodium thiosulfate $= N_2$?

Volume of sodium thiosulfate consumed $= V_2$ ml

$N_1 V_1 = N_2 V_2$

Potassium iodate $=$ Sodium thiosulfate

Normality of sodium thiosulfate $(N_2) = N_1 V_1 / V_2$

B. **Determination of copper sulfate:**

Factor

Each ml of 0.1 N $Na_2S_2O_3$ is equivalent to 0.02497 g of $CuSO_4.5H_2O$.

Weight of sample $= W$ g

Volume of sodium thiosulfate consumed $= V$ ml

$$\% \text{ purity of copper sulfate} = \frac{0.0249 \times V \times (N_2) \times 100}{W \times 0.1}$$

Result

The % purity of copper sulfate is ... %.

Judge yourself

1. Why acetic acid is added in copper sulfate titration?
2. Define the iodometric titration.
3. Why potassium thiocyanate is added in copper sulfate titration?
4. Why sodium thiosulfate is not a primary standard?

EXPERIMENT 30

Determination of potassium iodide

Potassium iodide occurs as colorless or white crystals, or a white crystalline powder. It is very soluble in water, soluble in ethanol, and practically insoluble in diethyl ether. It is slightly deliquescent in moist air.

Potassium iodide is an expectorant. It thins mucus secretions in the respiratory tract that may be caused by chronic respiratory problems such as asthma, chronic bronchitis, and emphysema. Potassium iodide is also used to protect the thyroid gland from radiation injury before and following administration of radioactive iodide (e.g. for diagnostic purposes) and in radiation emergencies (e.g. accidental exposure to radiation).

Experimental overview

Potassium iodide contains not less than 99% w/w of KI calculated with reference to the dried substance.

Potassium iodate oxidizes quantitatively iodides into iodine.

$$5KI + KIO_3 + 6HCl \longrightarrow KCl + 5ICl + 3H_2O$$

The liberated iodine reacts with excess of iodate in the presence of strong hydrochloric acid to form iodine monochloride (ICl).

$$2I_2 + KIO_3 + 6HCl \longrightarrow KCl + 5ICl + 3H_2O$$

In the titration, starch mucilage cannot be used as an indicator due to presence of strong hydrochloric acid which may be hydrolyzed, hence, chloroform is used. Iodine is more soluble in chloroform. The solution becomes colorless when whole iodine reacts with iodate.

Reagents required

1. 0.05 M KIO_3 solution. Dissolve about 10.7 g in KIO_3 in sufficient water and then make up the volume to 1 litre.
2. HCl.
3. Chloroform.

Procedure

Weigh accurately about 0.5 g of potassium iodide, dissolve in 10 ml of water and add 25 ml of hydrochloric acid and 5 ml of chloroform. Titrate it with 0.05 M potassium iodate until purple color disappears from the chloroform layer.

Observation and calculation

Weight of KI = W g

Volume of 0.05 KIO_3 consumed = V ml

Each ml of 0.05 M potassium iodate solution = 0.0166 g of KI.

$$\% \text{ purity} = \frac{0.0166 \times V \times 100}{W}$$

Result

The % purity of KI ... %.

Judge yourself

1. Why starch mucilage is not used as indicator in this titration?
2. Mention the uses of KI.
3. Why KI is added in redox iodometric titration even in the presence of sodium thiosulfate as a reducing agent?
4. Why concentrated hydrochloric acid is used?

EXPERIMENT 31

Determination of vitamin C

Vitamin C is an essential substance for maintaining good health and it is proved to be the agent which prevents scurvy. Most animals can synthesize their own vitamin C, but some, such as human, cannot. Owing to the increasing concern for one's health since the last century, vitamin C tablets have become the most popular supplement to normal diets.

Ascorbic acid

METHOD–I (DIRECT TITRATION WITH IODINE)

Experimental overview

Triiodide oxidizes vitamin C to form dehydroascorbic acid:

$$C_6H_8O_6 + I_3^- + H_2O \longrightarrow C_6H_6O_6 + 3I^- + 2H^+$$

As long as vitamin C is present in the solution, the triiodide is converted to the iodide ion very quickly. However, when all the vitamin C is oxidized, iodine and triiodide will be present, which react with starch to form a blue-black complex. The blue-black color is the endpoint of the titration.

Reagents required

1. **0.05 M iodine solution:** Weigh 36 g of potassium iodide into a 100 ml beaker. Weigh 14 g of iodine and add it into the same beaker. Add a few ml of distilled water and swirl for a few minutes until iodine is dissolved. Transfer iodine solution to a 1 L volumetric flask, making sure to rinse all traces of solution into the volumetric flask using distilled water. Make the solution up to the 1 L mark with distilled water.

2. **Starch indicator solution (0.5%):** Weigh 0.25 g of soluble starch and add it to 50 ml of near boiling water in a 100 ml conical flask. Stir to dissolve and cool before using.

Procedure

1. **Standardization of 0.05 M iodine solution:** Weigh accurately about 0.15 g of arsenic trioxide previously dried at 105°C for 1 hour and dissolve in 20 ml of 1 M sodium hydroxide solution by warming if necessary. Dilute with 40 ml of water, add 2 drops of methyl orange solution and add dilute HCl solution until the yellow color changed into pink color. Then add 2 g of NaHCO₃, dilute with 50 ml of water and add 3 ml of starch mucilage indicator. Slowly titrate with iodine solution until permanent blue color. Each ml of 0.05 M iodine solution is equivalent to 0.004948 g of arsenic trioxide.

   Chemical reaction : $As_2O_3 + 2H_2O \longrightarrow As_2O_5 + 4H^+ + 4e^-$

   $$As_2O_3 + 2I_2 + 2H_2O \longrightarrow As_2O_5 + 4H^+ + 4I^-$$

2. **Determination of ascorbic acid:** Weigh accurately about 0.1 g and dissolve in a mixture of 100 ml of freshly boiled and cooled water and 25 ml of dilute sulfuric acid. Immediately titrate with 0.05 M iodine using starch mucilage as indicator.

Observation and calculation

1. Calculation of molarity of iodine solution

$$\text{Molarity} = \frac{\text{Weight of As}_2O_3(g) \times 2}{197.7 \times \text{Vol. of iodine solution consumed (L)}}$$

Note: The factor 2 is required because each mole of As_2O_3 reacts with 2 moles of iodine (use above reaction).

197.7 is the molecular weight of arsenic trioxide.

2. Determination of ascorbic acid

Weight of ascorbic acid powder = W g

Volume of iodine consumed = V ml

1 mole of ascorbic acid = 1 mole of iodine

1000 ml of 1 M iodine = 1 M iodine = 1 ascorbic acid ($C_6H_8O_6$)

Each ml of 0.05 M iodine solution = 0.008806 g of $C_6H_8O_6$

$$\% \text{ purity of ascorbic acid} = \frac{0.008806 \times V \times \text{Molarity (cal.)}}{W \times \text{Molarity (given)}} \times 100 = ...\%$$

Result

The % purity of ascorbic acid is ... %.

METHOD–II (POTASSIUM IODATE METHOD)

Experimental view

Vitamin C is ascorbic acid, which is rapidly and quantitatively oxidized by iodine in acidic solution according to the following equation.

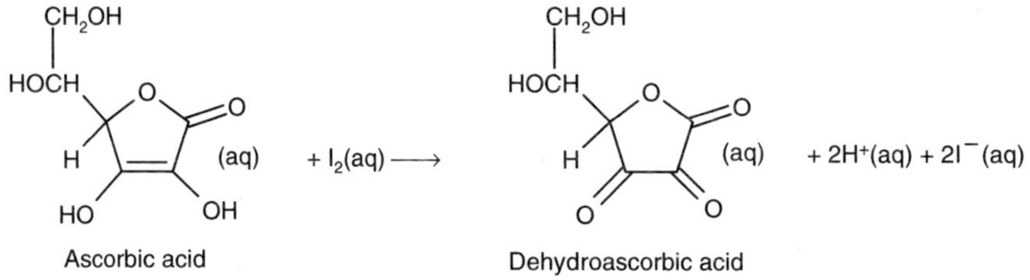

Ascorbic acid + I_2(aq) ⟶ Dehydroascorbic acid + 2H$^+$(aq) + 2I$^-$(aq)

The standard method for determination of ascorbic acid involves the direct titration of acidified sample with a standard iodine solution. But the low solubility of iodine makes this procedure less than ideal.

The proposed experiment avoids these difficulties by using the reaction between iodide (in excess) and iodate which generates a known excess quantity of iodine, and this excess iodine is back titrated with standard sodium thiosulfate solution.

The reactions are as follows:

$$IO_3^-(aq) + 5I^-(aq) + 6H^+(aq) \longrightarrow 3I_2(aq) + 3H_2O(l)$$

$$I_2(aq) + 2S_2O_3^{2-}(aq) \longrightarrow 2I^-(aq) + S_4O_6^{2-}(aq)$$

Reagents required

1. Vitamin C tablet.
2. Standard 0.01 M potassium iodate (KIO_3) solution. Weigh approximately 2.1 g (to the nearest 0.1 mg) of dried and reagent grade KIO_3. Transfer quantitatively to a 1000 ml volumetric flask. Initially, dissolve the KIO_3 in about 200 ml of distilled water. Dilute to the mark and mix thoroughly. Calculate the concentration of the KIO_3 solution.
3. Standard 0.060 M sodium thiosulfate solution. Dissolve 0.05 g sodium carbonate and 7.5 g sodium thiosulfate pentahydrate in water and dilute to 500 ml in a volumetric flask. This solid may be weighed on a top-loading balance, because the solution will be standardized against the potassium iodate solution. The sodium carbonate should be dissolved first to prevent the thiosulfate ion from experiencing an acidic environment.
4. Potassium iodide.
5. 0.5 M H_2SO_4 solution. Add 30 ml of concentrated sulfuric acid to 970 ml of water.
6. Freshly prepared starch solution. Weigh 0.25 g of soluble starch and add it to 50 ml of near boiling water in a 100 ml conical flask. Stir to dissolve and cool before using.

Procedure

1. **Standardization of sodium thiosulfate:**
   (a) Weigh accurately about 1.3 g of KIO_3 to prepare the 0.060 M KIO_3 solution and transfer to 250 ml volumetric flask. Dissolve in water and make up the volume.
   (b) Pipette 25.00 ml of the KIO_3 solution into a 250 ml Erlenmeyer flask.
   (c) Add 2 g of solid KI and 10 ml of 0.5 M H_2SO_4.
   (d) Immediately titrate with the thiosulfate solution until the solution has lost its initial reddish-brown color and has become pale yellow.
   (e) Add 2 ml of starch indicator and complete the titration until blue color disappear.

2. **Determination of ascorbic acid:**
   (a) Dissolve the vitamin C tablet provided (Roche Vitamin C effervescent tablet, claimed to contain 1 g of ascorbic acid) in about 150 ml of 0.5 M sulfuric acid.
   (b) Transfer the resulting solution to a clean volumetric flask and make up to 250 ml using distilled water.
   (c) Pipette 25.0 ml of the vitamin C solution into a conical flask and add to it 5 ml of 1 M potassium iodide solution. Then pipette 25.0 ml of the standard KIO_3 solution into the flask containing vitamin C and potassium iodide. The excess iodine is immediately back titrated with the standard sodium thiosulfate solution. Add a few drops of freshly prepared starch solution when the reaction mixture turns pale yellow and continue to titrate to the endpoint.

   Note:
   (i) Starch solution is used as an indicator. Iodine forms a complex with starch which is dark blue. The endpoint of the titration can be detected by the complete disappearance of the blue color. By knowing the total quantity of iodine formed, and the quantity left after

reaction with vitamin C, the amount of iodine reacted with the vitamin C can be calculated, hence the vitamin C concentration. The starch solution cannot be added earlier but only when the reaction mixture (iodine solution) fades to a straw color (pale yellow), by the time most of the iodine has been reduced. It is because with iodine is still in high concentration, it would form a blue-black precipitate complex with starch irreversibly which does not dissolve again easily even though there is an excess of thiosulfate, so iodine would be locked up and would not be free to react.

(ii) After the addition of sulfuric acid to the reaction mixture, titrations should be carried out immediately, because iodine can easily vaporize and escape from the solution, causing loss of reacting substance. Acidification of the vitamin C sample also serves to stabilize ascorbic acid, which will otherwise decompose.

Observation and calculation

Record your results into the following table.

Titration of vitamin C tablet with standard $Na_2S_2O_3$ solution

Titration	Trial	1	2	3
Final burette reading (ml)				
Initial burette reading (ml)				
Volume of $Na_2S_2O_3$ added (ml)				

Average vol. of $Na_2S_2O_3$ used =

Molecular weight of ascorbic acid (vitamin C) = 176

A. Total iodine mole generated from known volume of known concentration:

$$IO_3^- \text{ (aq)} + 5I^- \text{ (aq)} + 6H^+ \text{ (aq)} \longrightarrow 3I_2 \text{ (aq)} + 3H_2O \text{ (l)}$$

Standard solution   Excess

Ascorbic acid   Dehydroascorbic acid

From the stoichiometric calculation:

$$\frac{IO_3^- \text{ (mol)}}{1} = \frac{I_2 \text{ (mol)}}{3} = \frac{C_6H_8O_6 \text{ (mol)}}{3}$$

Known concentration 0.01 M   No. of moles of I_2 produced

Known volume 25 ml   can be calculated (3♥)

Hence, No. of moles of IO_3^- used

can be calculated (♥)

B. **Calculation of excess of unreacted iodine mole:**

$$I_2 \text{ (aq)} + \text{vitamin C} \longrightarrow \text{Dehydroascorbic acid} + 2H^+ \text{ (aq)} + 2I^- \text{ (aq)}$$

♦ (No. of moles of I_2 reacted with Vit. C).

$$2S_2O_3^{2-} \text{ (aq)} + I_2 \text{ (aq)} \longrightarrow 2I^- \text{ (aq)} + S_4O_6^{2-} \text{ (aq)}$$

Standard   Excess

solution

$$2S_2O_3^{2-} \equiv I_2 \sim S_2O_3^{2-} \equiv \frac{1}{2}I_2$$

No. of moles of $S_2O_3^{2-}$ used   No. of moles of excess I_2.

can be calculated (♣)   can be calculated (♣)

C. **Calculation of reacted iodine mole:**

No. of moles of I_2 (♦) reacted with vitamin C $= 3 \spadesuit - \dfrac{1}{2} \clubsuit$

D. **The content of ascorbic acid:**

No. of moles of vitamin C (in 25 ml solution) = ♦ (1 mole of I_2 = 1 mole of ascorbic acid)

250 ml of solution contains ♦ × 10 moles of ascorbic acid

One tablet of vitamin C contains ♦ × 10 moles of ascorbic acid

Mass (mg) of vitamin C per tablet ♦ × 10 × 176 g of ascorbic acid

Sample calculation

Average volume of $Na_2S_2O_3$ used = 8 ml

No. of moles of KIO_3 in 25 ml solution of 0.0110 M $KIO_3 = \dfrac{0.011 \times 25}{1000} = 0.00025$ moles

No. of moles of $I_2 = 3 \times 0.00025 = 0.00075$

No. of moles of $Na_2S_2O_3$ in 8 ml of 0.060 M $Na_2S_2O_3$ solution $= \dfrac{0.06}{1000} \times 8 = 0.00048$ moles

No. of moles of excess iodine $= \dfrac{1}{2} \times 0.00048 = 0.00024$ moles

No. of moles of I_2 reacted with vitamin C = 0.00075 – 0.00024 = 0.00051

Mass (in g) of vitamin C per tablet = 0.00051 × 10 × 176 = 0.897 of ascorbic acid

Potassium iodate method (IInd method) for ascorbic acid tablet

Procedure

1. Weigh one tablet (vitamin C content, <250 mg), powder it and dissolve in 50 ml of water.
2. Prepare to such sample.
3. Add 2 ml of 1 M KI solution, 2 ml of 1 M HCl solution and 1 ml of 2% starch solution.
4. Titrate the content with 0.025 M KIO_3 solution till blue-black colored complex appears.
5. Repeat this with second sample.

Note: *If the vitamin C content is more than 250 mg/tablet, then take one tablet, powder it and dissolve in sufficient water and then make up the volume to 100 ml. From this, pipet out 25 ml and do the same as done with low dose vitamin C tablet.*

Calculation

For low dose tablet (<250 mg/tablet)

Amount of vitamin C content/tablet = $V \times 0.025$ M $\times 3 \times 176 = \ldots$ mg/tablet

For high dose tablet (>250 mg/tablet)

Amount of vitamin C content/tablet = $V \times 0.025$ M $\times 3 \times 176 \times 100/25 = \ldots$ mg/tablet, where V is the volume of potassium iodate consumed in the titration of vitamin C content in tablet.

Judge yourself

1. What is the function of the starch solution? Why it has to be added only when the reaction mixture becomes pale yellow?
2. Why the titrations have to be carried out immediately after the addition of sulfuric acid?
3. Why the solution is acidified before titration?
4. Is KIO_3 a primary standard in this experiment? Why or why not? Give at least two reasons.
5. Sodium thiosulfate decomposes in an acidic environment. Write a balanced equation for this reaction.
6. 25.00 ml sample of orange drink with 2 g of KI and 25.00 ml of 0.0130 M KIO_3 added was back-titrated with a 0.0311 M sodium thiosulfate solution. The titration took 31.24 ml of thiosulfate. Calculate the ascorbic acid concentration in the orange drink in mg/ml.

EXPERIMENT 32

Determination of % purity of paracetamol by redox titration

Paracetamol (4–acetamidophenol) is a popular analgesic and an effective antipyretic The aim of this analytical procedure is to determine the % purity of paracetamol.

Experimental overview

Paracetamol on heating with sulfuric acid is hydrolysed into p-aminophenol and acetic acid. The p–aminophenol is oxidized into benzoquinone by ceric sulfate. The difference in two titrations indicates the amount required to oxidize the p-aminophenol liberated on hydrolysis of paracetamol.

| Paracetamol | p-Aminophenol | p-Benzoquinone |

Reagents required

1. **0.1 M ceric ammonium sulfate solution:** Dissolve 63.26 g of cerium ammonium sulfate in a mixture of 500 ml of water and 30 ml of sulfuric acid. Allow to cool and dilute to 1000.0 ml with water.
2. Sulfuric acid.
3. Ferroin indicator.

Procedure

1. **Standardization of 0.1 M ceric ammonium sulfate solution:** The standardization is based upon the oxidation of sodium arsenite by the ceric component of the salt, using ferroin as indicator.

$$NaAsO_2 + 2H_2O \longrightarrow NaH_2AsO_4 + 2H^+ + 4e$$
$$4[Ce^{4+} + e \longrightarrow Ce^{3+}]$$

Sodium arsenite is formed by dissolving the arsenic trioxide in NaOH solution. Accurately weigh about 0.2 g of arsenic trioxide and dissolve by gently heating in 15 ml of 0.2 M sodium hydroxide. Add to the clear solution 50 ml of sulfuric acid (~100 g/L) TS, 0.15 ml of a 2.5 mg/ml solution of osmium tetroxide in sulfuric acid (~100 g/L), and 0.1 ml of ferroin sulfate indicator. Titrate the solution with the ceric ammonium sulfate solution until red color disappears. Titrate slowly as the endpoint is approached.

2. **Determination of paracetamol:** Weigh accurately paracetamol (about 0.5 g) and transfer it into mixture of 1 M H_2SO_4 (50 ml) and water (10 ml). Boil the solution on water-bath for 1 hr. Cool, dilute with water to 100 ml. Pipette out 20 ml of this solution and transfer it into water (40 ml) containing 40 gm of crushed ice and 2 M HCl (15 ml) and ferroin indicator (0.1 ml) Titrate with 0.1 M ceric ammonium sulfate solution. Similarly, perform the blank titration.

Observation and calculation

Sample calculation

Molecular weight of arsenic trioxide = 197.84

Weight of arsenic trioxide = 0.1974 g (= 197.4 mg)

Volume of ceric ammonium sulfate = 30.00 ml

M moles of As_2O_3 = weight (mg)/197.84 [= 198.4/197.84] = 1.002 m moles

From the above equation:

4 moles of Ce^{4+} = 1 mole of $NaASO_2$

Hence, 1 mole of $NaAsO_2$ (or As_2O_3) = $4Ce^{4+}$

1.002 M moles of $NaAsO_2$ (or As_2O_3) = 4 × 1.002 = 4.008 m moles Ce^{4+}

Molarity of Ce^{4+} = (m mol Ce^{4+}/ml ceric ammonium sulfate [= 4.008/30] = 0.133 M

Determination of paracetamol:

Molecular weight of paracetamol = 151.16

Weight of powder = W g

Volume of 0.1 M ceric ammonium sulfate solution consumed (in sample) = V_1

Volume of 0.1 M ceric ammonium sulfate solution consumed (in blank) = V_2 ml

Difference between sample and blank titrations = $V_1 - V_2 = V$ ml

From the above equation:

2 moles of ceric ammonium sulfate = 1 mole of $C_8H_9NO_2$

Each ml of 0.1 M ceric ammonium sulphate solution = 0.00756 g of paracetamol.

V ml of 0.1 M ceric sulfate solution = 0.00756 (V) g of $C_8H_9NO_2$

W g of sample (dissolved in 100 ml) is equivalent to 0.00756 × V × 5 g of $C_8H_9NO_2$

(where 5 is the dilution factor)

$$\% \text{ purity of paracetamol} = \frac{0.00756 \times V \times \text{molarity (cal.)}}{W \times \text{molarity (given)}} \times 100 = ...\%$$

Result

The % purity of paracetamol is ... %.

Judge yourself

1. What is the basis of estimation of paracetamol?
2. Why estimation of paracetamol in tablet is not recommended by redox titration in IP?
3. Why blank titration is carried out?

Non-aqueous Titrations

Introduction

Non-aqueous titration is the titration of substances dissolved in non-aqueous solvents. It is the most common titrimetric procedure used in pharmacopoeial assays and serves a double purpose: it is suitable for the titration of very weak acids and very weak bases, and it provides a solvent in which organic compounds are soluble.

The most commonly used procedure is the titration of organic bases with perchloric acid in *anhydrous* acetic acid.

The theory is that water behaves as both a weak acid and a weak base; thus, in an aqueous environment, it can compete effectively with very weak acids or bases with regard to proton donation or acceptance, respectively, as shown below:

$$H_2O + H^+ \rightleftharpoons H_3O^+$$

Competes with

$$RNH_2 + H^+ \rightleftharpoons RNH_3^+$$

or

$$H_2O + B \rightleftharpoons OH^- + BH^+$$

Competes with

$$ROH + B \rightleftharpoons RO^- + BH^+.$$

The effect of this is that the inflection in the titration curves for very weak acids and very weak bases is small, because they approach the pH limits in water of 14 or 0 respectively, thus making endpoint detection relatively more difficult.

A general rule is that bases with $pK_a < 7$ or acids with $pK_a > 7$ cannot be determined accurately in aqueous solution.

Substances which are either too weakly basic or too weakly acidic to give sharp endpoints in aqueous solution can often be titrated in non-aqueous solvents. The reactions which occur during many non-aqueous titrations can be explained by means of the concepts of the Brønsted-Lowry theory. According to this theory, an acid is a proton donor, i.e. a substance which tends to dissociate to yield a proton, and a base is proton acceptor, i.e. a substance which tends to combine with a proton. When an acid HB dissociates it yields a proton together with the conjugate base B of the acid:

$$\underset{\text{acid}}{HB} \rightleftharpoons \underset{\text{proton}}{H^+} + \underset{\text{base}}{B^-}$$

Alternatively, the base B will combine with a proton to yield the conjugate acid HB of the base B, for every base has its conjugate acid and, every acid has its conjugate base.

It follows from these definitions that an acid may be either:

- an electrically neutral molecule, e.g. HCl, or
- a positively charged cation, e.g. $C_6H_5NH_3^+$, or
- a negatively charged anion, e.g. HSO_4^-.

A base may be either:

- an electrically neutral molecule, e.g. $C_6H_5NH_2$, or
- an anion, e.g. Cl^-.

Substances which are potentially acidic can function as acids only in the presence of a base to which they can donate a proton. Conversely basic properties do not become apparent unless an acid also is present.

Non-aqueous solvents used

Aprotic solvents are neutral, chemically inert substances such as benzene and chloroform. They do not react with either acids or bases and therefore do not favor ionization. The fact that picric acid gives a colorless solution in benzene which becomes yellow on adding aniline shows that picric acid is not dissociated in benzene solution and also that in the presence of the base aniline it functions as an acid, the development of yellow color being due to formation of the picrate ion.

Protophilic solvents are basic in character and react with acids to form solvated protons.

$$HB + Sol. \rightleftharpoons Sol.H^+ + B^-$$

Acid + Basic solvent $\rightleftharpoons$ Solvated proton + Conjugate base of acid

A weakly basic solvent has less tendency than a strongly basic one to accept a proton. Similarly a weak acid has less tendency to donate protons than a strong acid. As a result a strong acid such as perchloric acid exhibits more strongly acidic properties than a weak acid such as acetic acid when dissolved in a weakly basic solvent. On the other hand, all acids tend to become indistinguishable in strength when dissolved in strongly basic solvents owing to the greater affinity of strong bases for protons. This is called the leveling effect. Strong bases are leveling solvents for acids, weak bases are differentiating solvents for acids.

Protogenic solvents are acidic substances, e.g. sulfuric acid. They exert a leveling effect on bases.

Amphiprotic solvents have both protophilic and protogenic properties. Examples are water, acetic acid and the alcohols. They are dissociated to a slight extent. The dissociation of acetic acid, which is frequently used as a solvent for titration of basic substances, is shown in the equation below:

$$CH_3COOH \rightleftharpoons H^+ + CH_3COO^-$$

Here, the acetic acid is functioning as an acid. If a very strong acid such as perchloric acid is dissolved in acetic acid, the latter can function as a base and combine with protons donated by the perchloric acid to form protonated acetic acid, an onium ion:

$$HClO_4 \rightleftharpoons H^+ + ClO_4^-$$

$$CH_3COOH + H^+ \rightleftharpoons CH_3COOH_2^+ \text{ (onium ion)}$$

Since the $CH_3COOH_2^+$ ion readily donates its proton to a base, a solution of perchloric acid in glacial acetic acid functions as a strongly acidic solution.

Acidimetry in non-aqueous titrations

For analysis, weak bases are dissolved in such solvent system to eliminate as far as possible the competing reaction of water for the proton besides enhancing the strength of the basic species.

For example, weak base, such as pyridine, is dissolved in acetic acid, the acetic acid exerts its levelling effect and enhances the basic properties of the pyridine. It is possible, therefore, to titrate a solution of a weak base in acetic acid with perchloric acid in acetic acid.

$$HClO_4 + CH_3COOH \rightleftharpoons CH_3COOH_2^+ + ClO_4^-$$

$$C_5H_5N + CH_3COOH \rightleftharpoons C_5H_5NH^+ + CH_3COO^-$$

$$CH_3COOH_2^+ + CH_3COO^- \rightleftharpoons 2CH_3COOH$$

The overall reaction:

$$HClO_4 + C_5H_5N \rightleftharpoons C_5H_5NH^+ + ClO_4^-$$

Titration of halogen acid salts of bases

The halide ions, chloride, bromide and iodide, are too weakly basic to react quantitatively with acetous perchloric acid. Addition of mercuric acetate (which is undissociated in acetic acid solution) to a halide salt replaces the halide ion by an equivalent quantity of acetate ion, which is a strong base in acetic acid.

$$2R.NH_2.HCl \rightleftharpoons 2RNH_3^+ + 2Cl^-$$

$$(CH_3COO)_2Hg \text{ (undissociated)} + 2Cl^- \rightleftharpoons HgCl_2 \text{ (undissociated)} + 2CH_3COO^-$$

$$2CH_3COOH_2^+ + 2CH_3COO^- \rightleftharpoons 4CH_3COOH$$

Alkalimetry in non-aqueous titrations

The weakly acidic pharmaceutical substances may be titrated effectively by making use of a suitable non-aqueous solvent with a sharp endpoint. The wide spectrum of such organic compounds include: anhydride, acids, amino acids, acid halides, enols (viz. barbiturates), xanthenes, sulphonamides, phenols, imides and lastly the organic salts of inorganic acids.

EXPERIMENT 33

Determination of chloroquine phosphate content in tablet

Chloroquine phosphate contains not less than 98.5 percent and not more than the equivalent of 101.0 per cent of N^4-(7-chloroquinolin-4-yl)-N^1,N^1-diethylpentane-1,4-diamine bis (dihydrogen phosphate), calculated with reference to the dried substance.

It is available as white or almost white, crystalline powder, hygroscopic, freely soluble in water, very slightly soluble in alcohol and in methanol. It exists in 2 forms, one of which melts at about 195°C and the other at about 218°C.

Chloroquine phosphate

Experimental overview

Chloroquine is a weak base so it is titrated with standard perchloric acid in glacial acetic acid.

Reagents required

1. 0.1 M $HClO_4$ solution. To 900 ml of glacial acetic acid add 8.5 ml of perchloric acid, mix, add 30 ml of acetic anhydride, dilute to 1000 ml with glacial acetic acid, mix and allow to stand for 24 hours.
2. Crystal violet indicator. Dissolve 0.2 g of crystal violet in 100 ml of acetic acid.
3. Glacial acetic acid.
4. Acetic anhydride.

Procedure

1. **Standardization of perchloric acid:** Weigh accurately about dissolve 0.35 g of potassium hydrogen phthalate (KHP) in 50 ml of anhydrous acetic acid, warming gently if necessary. Allow to cool protected from air and titrate with perchloric acid solution using 0.05 ml of crystal violet solution as indicator. Each ml of 0.1 M perchloric acid solution is equivalent to 20.42 mg of $C_8H_5KO_4$.

2. **Determination of chloroquine phosphate:**
   (i) Weigh accurately 20 tablets and powder them. Find out the average weight of tablet.

(ii) Transfer a quantity of powder equivalent to 0.5 g of chloroquine phosphate in a separating funnel, add 20 ml of 1 M NaOH solution and extract with four quantities of chloroform, each 25 ml. Filter the combined extract through glass fiber paper previously moistened with solvent. Evaporate the chloroform to get dried residue.

(iii) Dissolve in 40 ml of anhydrous acetic acid and titrate with 0.1 M perchloric acid determining the endpoint potentiometrically or with the use of crystal violet indicator.

Observation and calculation

1. **Determination of molarity of perchloric acid:**

$$\text{Molarity of HClO}_4 \text{ solution} = \frac{\text{Weight of KHP (g)}}{204 \times \text{Volume of HClO}_4 \text{ solution (L)}}$$

where 204 is the molecular weight of KHP.

2. **Determination of chloroquine phosphate:**

Weight of tablet powder = W g

Average weight of tablet = W_1 g

Volume of 0.1 M HClO$_4$ solution consumed = V ml

From the equation:

1 mole of chloroquine phosphate = 2HClO$_4$

1000 ml of 1.0 M HClO$_4$ solution = 257.9 g of C$_{18}$H$_{32}$ClN$_3$O$_8$P$_2$.

Each ml of 0.1 M perchloric acid solution = 0.02579 gm of C$_{18}$H$_{32}$ClN$_3$O$_8$P$_2$.

$$\text{The content of chloroquine phosphate in tablet} = \frac{0.02017 \times V \times \text{Molarity (cal)}}{0.1 \,(\text{molarity given}) \times W} \times W_1 = \text{.... g.}$$

Result

The average weight tablet is found to contain .... g of chloroquine phosphate.

Judge yourself

1. What is the basis of titration of chloroquine phosphate with perchloric acid?
2. Give the reaction involved in this titration.
3. What is the pH range of crystal violet indicator?
4. What is the % purity of perchloric acid?

EXPERIMENT 34

Determination of % purity of diclofenac sodium

Diclofenac sodium, 2-[2,6-dichlorophenyl)-amino] benzene acetic acid monosodium salt, is a nonsteroidal anti-inflammatory drug with potent activity and outstanding tolerability in the treatment of rheumatic disease. It is also used as an analgesic and antipyretic. This phenylacetic acid derivative acts as an inhibitor of hyaluronidase, prostaglandins synthesis and platelet aggregation. Other commonly used salts of diclofenac are those of potassium and diethylammonium salt. Diclofenac is presented as tablets (enteric coated, controlled release), creams and injectables.

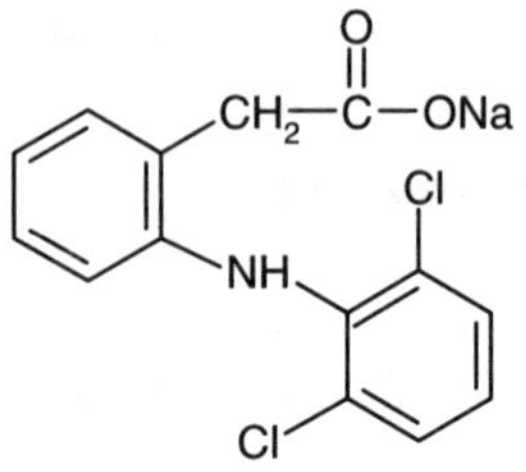

Diclofenac sodium

Experimental overview

It is a weak base, hence titrated with acetous perchloric acid using crystal violet as indicator.

Reagents required

1. 0.1 M $HClO_4$ solution. To 900 ml of glacial acetic acid, add 8.5 ml of perchloric acid, mix, add 30 ml of acetic anhydride, dilute to 1000 ml with glacial acetic acid, mix and allow to stand for 24 hours.
2. Potassium hydrogen phthalate.
3. Crystal violet indicator. Dissolve 0.2 g of crystal violet in 100 ml of acetic acid.
4. Glacial acetic acid.
5. Acetic anhydride.

Procedure

1. **Standardization of 0.1 M $HClO_4$ solution:** Weigh accurately about 350 mg of potassium hydrogen phthalate (KHP) and dissolve in 50 ml of anhydrous acetic acid with gentle warming gently (if necessary). Allow to cool protected from air and titrate with perchloric acid solution using 0.05 ml of crystal violet solution as indicator. Each ml of 0.1 M perchloric acid = 20.42 mg of $C_8H_5KO_4$.

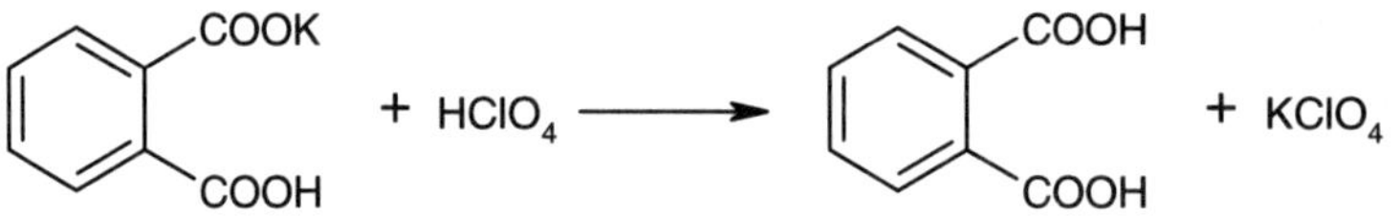

Note : Restandardize before use. Store in amber bottle with well-fitted suitable stoppers which prevent access to atmospheric carbon dioxide. Discard the solution after 30 days.

2. **Determination of diclofenac sodium:**
   (i) Weigh accurately about 0.2 g of diclofenac sodium and dissolve in 50 ml of glacial acetic acid.
   (ii) Add few drops crystal violet indicator and titrate with 0.1 M $HClO_4$ solution until green color.
   (iii) Similarly, perform a blank titration.

Observation and calculation

(i) **Standardization of perchloric acid:**

$$\text{Molarity of perchloric acid} = \frac{W(g)}{204 \times V \text{ (in litre)}}$$

where V = Volume of perchloric acid consumed in ml
W = Weight of potassium hydrogen phthalate in g
204 is the molecular weight of KHP

(ii) **Determination of diclofenac sodium:**
Molecular weight of diclofenac sodium = 318.14
Weight of sample = W g
Volume of 0.1 M $HClO_4$ consumed in diclofenac sodium titration = V_1 ml
Volume of 0.1 M $HClO_4$ consumed in blank titration = V_2 ml
Difference = $V_1 - V_2 = V$ ml
1 mole of diclofenac sodium = 1 mole of $HClO_4$ = 1000 ml of 1 M $HClO_4$
Hence, each ml of 0.1 M perchloric acid solution = 0.03181 g of $C_{14}H_{10}Cl_2NNaO_2$
The % of diclofenac sodium present in the sample is given by:

$$\% \text{ of diclofenac sodium} = \frac{0.03181 \times V \times \text{Molarity (cal.)}}{\text{Molarity (given)} \times W} \times 100 = ...\%$$

Result

The % of diclofenac sodium in sample is found to be ....%.

Judge yourself

1. Why acetic anhydride is added in the preparation of standard perchloric acid?
2. Why % of perchloric acid is low, about 70%?
3. Give the reactions involved in this titration.

EXPERIMENT 35

Determination of % purity of methyldopa

Methyldopa is an antihypertensive drug. Methyldopa, the L-isomer of alpha-methyldopa, is levo–3-(3,4-dihydroxyphenyl)-2-methylalanine. Its empirical formula is $C_{10}H_{13}NO_4$, with a molecular weight of 211.22, and its structural formula is:

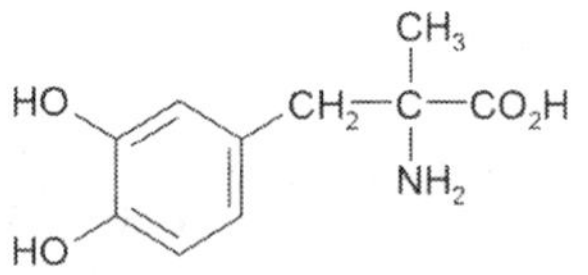

Methyldopa is a white to yellowish white, odorless fine powder, and is soluble in water. It is supplied as tablets, for oral use, in three strengths: 125 mg, 250 mg, or 500 mg of methyldopa per tablet.

Experimental overview

It is a weak base and so titrated with standard perchloric acid in glacial acetic acid. The reaction between methyldopa and perchloric acid is expressed by the following equation.

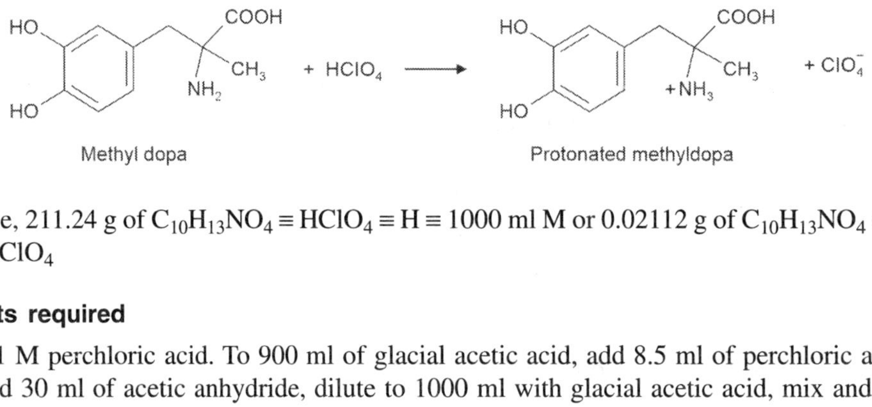

Methyl dopa   Protonated methyldopa

Hence, 211.24 g of $C_{10}H_{13}NO_4 \equiv HClO_4 \equiv H \equiv 1000$ ml M or 0.02112 g of $C_{10}H_{13}NO_4 \equiv 1$ ml of 0.1 M $HClO_4$

Reagents required

1. 0.1 M perchloric acid. To 900 ml of glacial acetic acid, add 8.5 ml of perchloric acid, mix, add 30 ml of acetic anhydride, dilute to 1000 ml with glacial acetic acid, mix and allow to stand for 24 hours.
2. Anhydrous formic acid.
3. Glacial acetic acid.
4. Dioxane.
5. Crystal violet indicator.

Procedure

1. **Standardization of 0.1 M perchloric acid solution:** Weigh accurately about 350 mg of potassium hydrogen phthalate (KHP) and dissolve in 50 ml of anhydrous acetic acid with gentle warming (if necessary). Allow to cool protected from air and titrate with perchloric acid solution using 0.05 ml of crystal violet solution as indicator. Each ml of 0.1 M perchloric acid = 20.42 mg of $C_8H_5KO_4$.

2. **Determination of methyldopa in tablet:**
   (i) Weigh accurately about 0.2 g of sample and dissolve in a mixture of 15 ml of anhydrous formic acid, 30 ml of glacial acetic acid and 30 ml of dioxane.
   (ii) Add 0.1 ml of crystal violet solution and titrate with 0.1 M perchloric acid until green color.
   (iii) Perform a blank determination and make any necessary correction.

Observation and calculation

1. Calculation of molarity of perchloric acid

$$\text{Molarity} = \frac{W(g)}{204 \times V \text{ (L)}}$$

where V = Volume of perchloric acid consumed in litre
W = Weight of potassium hydrogen phthalate in g
204 is the molecular weight of KHP

2. Determination of methyldopa
   Molecular wt. of methyldopa = 211
   Weight of sample = W g
   Volume of 0.1 M $HClO_4$ consumed = V ml
   Each ml of 0.1 N perchloric acid solution = 0.02112 g of $C_{10}H_{13}NO_4$
   The % of methyldopa present in the sample is given by:

$$\text{\% of methyldopa in sample} = \frac{0.0211 \times V \times \text{Molarity (cal)}}{\text{Molarity (given)} \times W} \times 100 = \text{....\%}$$

Result

The % of methyldopa in sample is found to be ....%.

Judge yourself

1. Give the reaction involved in the titration of methyldopa.
2. Mention the other methods to determine % purity of methyldopa.

EXPERIMENT 36

Determination of ephedrine HCl content in tablet

Ephedrine HCl is also an expectorant bronchodilator. It is taken for the temporary relief of shortness of breath, tightness of chest, and wheezing due to bronchial asthma. It also helps loosen mucus and thin bronchial secretions to drain bronchial tubes and make cough more productive.

Ephedrine

Experimental overview

It is difficult to titrate halogen salt directly with acetous perchloric acid because there is no much difference in the proton attracting capabilities of the halide ion and perchlorate anions in glacial acetic acid. Therefore, the reaction does not proceed toward completion. Hence, mercuric acetate is added to ephedrine chloride to replace an equivalent amount of acetate ion which is readily protonated. Mercuric chloride remains undissociated in glacial acetic acid.

$$2HClO_4 + 2CH_3COOH \longrightarrow 2CH_3COOH_2^+ + 2ClO_4^-$$

$$\underset{\text{Ephedrine HCl}}{2C_{10}H_{15}N^+HOCl^-} + \underset{\text{Mercuric acetate}}{(Ac)_2Hg} \longrightarrow 2C_{10}H_{15}N + HO.Ac + HgCl_2$$

$$CH_3COO^- + CH_3COOH_2^+ \longrightarrow 2CH_3COOH$$

$$2C_{10}H_{15}N + HO.Ac + 2CH_3COOH_2^+ \longrightarrow 2C_{10}H_{10}N^+HO + 4CH_3COOH$$

The overall reaction:

$$2C_{10}H_{15}N^+HOCl^- + (Ac)_2Hg + 2HClO_4 \longrightarrow 2C_{10}H_{10}N^+H + AcOH + 2ClO_4^- + HgCl_2$$

Reagents required

1. 0.1 M solution of HClO₄ solution. Dissolve 8.5 ml of 72% HClO₄ in about 900 ml glacial acetic acid with constant stirring, add about 30 ml acetic anhydride and make up the volume (1000 ml) with glacial acetic acid and keep the mixture for 24 hour.
   Acetic anhydride absorbed all the water from HClO₄ and glacial acetic acid and renders the solution virtually anhydrous. HClO₄ must be well diluted with glacial acetic acid before adding acetic anhydride because reaction between HClO₄ and acetic anhydride is explosive.
2. Crystal violet solution (0.2% w/v in acetic acid).
3. Mercuric acetate solution (5%w/v in acetic acid).
4. Glacial acetic acid.
5. Acetic anhydride.
6. Potassium hydrogen phthalate.

Procedure

1. **Standardization of the above prepared 0.1 M HClO₄ solution:** Weigh about 0.5 g of potassium acid phthalate (KHP), add 25 ml of glacial acetic acid and add few drops of 5% w/v crystal violet in glacial acetic acid as indicator. Titrate the solution with 0.1 M HClO₄ solution till blue green color appears.

Each ml of 0.1 N $HClO_4$ solution = 0.020414 g of potassium acid phthalate.

2. **Determination of ephedrine HCl content:** Weigh accurately 20 tablets and find out the average weight of tablet. Grind the tablets to fine powder. Weigh accurately a quantity of powder equivalent to about 0.15 g of ephedrine hydrochloride, add glacial acetic acid (30 ml), mercuric acetate solution (10 ml) and crystal violet solution (0.1 ml) to it. Gently warm the solution, cool and titrate with 0.1 M perchloric acid until the violet color changes to green blue. Perform a blank titration in the same way.

Observation and calculation

1. **Standardization of 0.1 M $HClO_4$ solution:**

$$\text{Molarity} = \frac{W(g)}{204 \times V \text{ (L)}}$$

where V = Volume of perchloric acid consumed in litre

W = Weight of potassium hydrogen phthalate in g

204 is the molecular weight of KHP

2. **Determination of ephedrine HCl:**

Molecular wt. of ephedrine HCl = 201.7

Weight of tablet powder = W g

Average weight of tablet = W_1 g

Volume of 0.1 M $HClO_4$ solution consumed = V ml

From the equation:

1 mole of $C_{10}H_{15}NO.HCl.$ = Cl^- + CH_3COO^- = $HClO_4$

1000 ml of 1.0 M $HClO_4$ solution = 201.7 g of ephedrine HCl

Each ml of 0.1 M perchloric acid solution = 0.02017 gm of $C_{10}H_{15}NO.HCl.$

$$\text{The content of ephedrine HCl in tablet} = \frac{0.02017 \times V \times \text{Molarity (cal)}}{0.1 \text{ (molarity given)} \times W} \times W_1 = \text{.... g}$$

Result

The average weight tablet is found to contain .... g of ephedrine HCl.

Judge yourself

1. Why mercuric acetate is added in this titration?
2. What is use of ephedrine HCl?
3. How pseudoephedrine differs from ephedrine?
4. How many chiral centres exist in ephedrine?

EXPERIMENT 37

Determination of chlorpromazine HCl content in tablet

Reference: Henry A Okeri, Peter O Alonge and Emadoye Etareri, International Journal of Health Research, 1(1), 21–26 (2008).

Chlorpromazine (10-[3-dimethylaminopropyl] phenothiazine) belongs to the primary chemical group of antipsychotic agents known as the phenothiazines. It has an aliphatic side chain and is referred to as an atypical phenothiazine with a low to moderate potency antipsychotic action. Apart from its antipsychotic activity, where it is used as a tranquilizer and maintenance therapy to prevent acute relapse in chronic schizophrenic patients, chlorpromazine is also used for the treatment of vomiting and vertigo because of its sedative and extrapyramidal effects.

—Cl

•HCl

$(CH_2)_3N(CH_3)_2$

Chlorpromazine HCl

Experimental overview

The determination of the chlorpromazine hydrochloride content is based on non-aqueous titration. Glacial acetic acid is used as the non-aqueous solvent and equivalence point is determined using visual indicators and potentiometer. Some of the official monographs (International Pharmacopeia, British Pharmacopoeia and United States Pharmacopoeia) specify perchloric acid titration for the assay of chlorpromazine HCl. The addition of mercuric acetate in the non-aqueous titrimetric method is based on the principle of removing the chloride counter ion so as to prevent the interference of the halide ion released by the titrant (acetous perchloric acid). The addition of mercuric acetate (which is undissociated in acetic acid) replaces the halide ion in chlorpromazine with a quantitative acetate ion which is a strong base in acetic acid. An intense red-colored oxidation product is formed when ascorbic acid is not added. This makes endpoint detection with visual indicators to be difficult.

Reagents required

1. 0.1 M solution of $HClO_4$ solution. Dissolve 8.5 ml of 72% $HClO_4$ in about 900 ml glacial acetic acid with constant stirring, add about 30 ml acetic anhydride and make up the volume (1000 ml) with glacial acetic acid and keep the mixture for 24 hour.
   Acetic anhydride absorbs all the water from $HClO_4$ and glacial acetic acid and renders the solution virtually anhydrous. $HClO_4$ must be well diluted with glacial acetic acid before adding acetic anhydride because reaction between $HClO_4$ and acetic anhydride is explosive.
2. Crystal violet solution (0.2% w/v in acetic acid).
3. Mercuric acetate solution (5% w/v in acetic acid).
4. Glacial acetic acid.
5. Acetic anhydride.

Procedure

1. **Standardization of the above prepared 0.1 M HClO₄ solution:** Weigh about 0.5 g of potassium acid phthalate (KHP) add 25 ml of glacial acetic acid and add few drops of 5% w/v crystal violet in glacial acetic acid as indicator. Titrate the solution with 0.1 M HClO₄ solution till blue green color appears.

Each ml of 0.1 N HClO₄ = 0.020414 g of potassium acid phthalate.

2. **Determination of chlorpromazine HCl in tablet:**
   (i) Weigh accurately twenty tablets and reduce to fine powder.
   (ii) From the powdered drug, take an amount equivalent to 0.35 g of chlorpromazine HCl and transfer into a 250 ml conical flask containing 50 ml of glacial acetic acid.
   (iii) Shake the mixture and add 10 ml of 5% w/v mercuric acetate, 2 g of ascorbic acid and 2 drops of 0.2% w/v crystal violet indicator.
   (iv) Stir the solution for 15 min with a magnetic stirrer and then titrate with 0.1 M acetous perchloric acid to a blue endpoint.
   (v) Do all the steps in triplicates.

Note: Ascorbic acid prevents the development of color and so allows the determination of endpoint by crystal violet indicator.

Observation and calculation

1. **Standardization of 0.1 M HClO₄ solution:**

$$\text{Molarity} = \frac{W(g)}{204 \times V \text{ (L)}}$$

where V = Volume of perchloric acid consumed in litre
   W = Weight of potassium hydrogen phthalate in g
   204 is the molecular weight of KHP

2. **Determination of chlorpromazine HCl:**
   Molecular weight of chlorpromazine HCl = 355.78
   Weight of tablet powder = W g
   Average weight of tablet = W_1 g
   Volume of 0.1 M HClO₄ solution consumed = V ml

   From the equation:
   1 mole of $C_{17}H_{19}ClN_2S.HCl = Cl^- + CH_3COO^- = HClO_4$
   1000 ml of 1.0 M HClO₄ solution = 355.3 g of chlorpromazine HCl
   1 ml of 0.1 M HClO₄ solution = 0.03553 g of chlorpromazine HCl

   The content of chlorpromazine HCl in tablet = $\dfrac{0.03553 \times V \times \text{Molarity (cal.)}}{0.1 \times W} \times W_1 = \ldots.$ g

Result

The average weight tablet is found to contain .... g of chlorpromazine HCl.

Judge yourself

1. Why ascorbic acid is added?
2. How chlorpromazine HCl acts as antipsychotic drug?
3. What is the basis of titrations of amines?

EXPERIMENT 38

Determination of % purity of ethosuximide

Experimental overview

Ethosuximide is a weak acid so titrated with standard sodium methoxide solution in dimethyl formamide which enhances its acidity.

Ethosuximide   Sodium salt of Ethosuximide

Reagents required

1. **0.1 M sodium methoxide solution:** Cool in ice-water 150 ml of methanol contained in a 1000 ml volumetric flask, and add, in small portions, about 2.5 g of freshly cut sodium metal. When the metal has dissolved, add toluene to make 1000 ml, and mix. Store preferably in the reservoir of an automatic delivery buret suitably protected from carbon dioxide and moisture
2. Dimethylformamide.
3. Azo-violet (0.1% w/v in DMF).

Procedure

1. **Standardization of above prepared 0.1 M sodium methoxide solution:** Accurately weigh about 400 mg of primary standard benzoic acid, and dissolve in 80 ml of dimethylformamide in a flask. Add 3 drops of a 1 in 100 solution of thymol blue in dimethylformamide, and titrate with the sodium methoxide to a blue endpoint. Correct for the volume of the sodium methoxide solution consumed by 80 ml of the dimethylformamide, and calculate the molarity. Sodium methoxide is standardized by primary standard benzoic acid in DMF which enhances its acidity. The reaction are as follows:

$$C_6H_5COOH + HCON(CH_3)_2 \longrightarrow HCON^+H(CH_3)_2 + C_6H_5COO^-$$

$$CH_3ONa \longrightarrow CH_3O^- + Na^+$$

$$HCON^+H(CH_3)_2 + CH_3O^- \longrightarrow HCON(CH_3)_2 + CH_3OH$$

Overall reaction is:

$$C_6H_5COOH + CH_3ONa \longrightarrow C_6H_5COONa + CH_3OH$$

Each ml of 0.1 M sodium methoxide is equivalent to 0.01221 g of benzoic acid.

Notes:

(1) To eliminate any turbidity that may form following dilution with toluene, add methanol (25 to 30 ml usually suffices) until the solution is clear.
(2) Restandardize the solution frequently.

2. **Determination of ethosuximide:**

(i) Weigh accurately about 0.2 g of the sample and dissolve in 50 ml of dimethylformamide.

(ii) Add 2 drops of azo-violet solution and titrate with 0.1 N sodium methoxide to a deep blue endpoint, taking precautions to prevent absorption of atmospheric carbon dioxide.

(iii) Perform a blank determination and make any necessary correction.

Each ml of 0.1 N sodium methoxide is equivalent to 0.01412 g of $C_7H_{11}NO_2$.

Observation and calculation

1. **Determination of molarity of sodium methoxide solution:**

$$\text{Molarity} = \frac{\text{Weight of benzoic acid (g)}}{122 \times \text{Volume of } CH_3ONa \text{ consumed (L)}}$$

122 is the molecular weight of benzoic acid

2. **Determination of ethosuximide:**

Weight of sample = W g

Volume of 0.1 M $HClO_4$ consumed = V ml

141.17 g $C_7H_{11}NO_2 \equiv$ NaOMe $\equiv$ H $\equiv$ 1000 ml M

Each ml of 0.1 M perchloric acid solution = 0.0141 g $C_7H_{11}NO_2$

The % of ethosuximide present in the sample is given by:

$$\% \text{ of ethosuximide in sample} = \frac{0.0141 \times V \times \text{Molarity (cal)}}{\text{Molarity (given)} \times W} \times 100 = ...\%$$

Result

The % of ethosuximide in the given sample is found to be ....%.

Judge yourself

1. Why toluene is used to prepare the sodium methoxide solution?
2. Why methanol is cooled to prepare the standard sodium methoxide solution?

Diazotization Titration or Nitrite Titration

Introduction

Diazotization is used for the analysis of aromatic compounds containing an amino group in the molecules. It is based on the reaction between aromatic primary amine ($-NH_2$), and nitrous acid (HONO), at low temperature (below 10°C).

$NaNO_2$ is generally used in direct method of diazotization. It gives HNO_2 in acidic solution. Many aromatic primary amine with free $-NH_2$ group can be analyzed quantitatively by measuring the volume of $NaNO_2$ solution required to convert them into diazonium salts. The typical reaction of diazotization reaction in presence of HCl is given as:

$$NaNO_2 + HCl \longrightarrow HONO + NaCl$$
$$ArNH_2 + HONO + HCl \longrightarrow ArN_2^+Cl^- + 2H_2O$$
$$\text{Aryldiazonium chloride}$$

When all the aromatic amine has reacted with $NaNO_2$ then slight excess of $NaNO_2$ added to the solution under test, converted to HONO that remain in the solution and can be detected by the starch paper or paste as an external indicator. This appearance of free HNO_2 in solution indicates that diazotization reaction is complete and equivalence point is attained.

Starch iodide paper or paste is the starch solution plus equal volume of 5% KI solution in H_2O. Starch iodide paste reacts with reaction mixture as follows:

$$KI + HCl \longrightarrow HI + KCl$$
$$2HI + 2HONO \longrightarrow I_2\uparrow + 2NO + 2H_2O$$
$$\text{(excess)}$$
$$I_2 + Starch \longrightarrow \text{Blue color}$$

The liberated I_2 reacts with starch to give blue color. The diazotization proceeds quantitatively only in presence of inorganic acid. It is important to check the acidity at the end of the titration.

If there is no excess of acid present, starch-iodide paper will not detect excess HNO_2 and so will not indicate the endpoint.

Conditions for diazotization

1. Rate of titration.
2. Temperature of the solution.
(1) **Rate of titration:** Different amino compound react with HONO at different rates. $NaNO_2$ added from the burette needs time to react with amino group accumulating in the solution.

Amines are classified as rapidly or slowly diazotisable depending on the rate of conversion into azo compounds. Slow diazotisable compounds include compounds that contain SO_2NH_2 groups, nitrous oxide group, or carboxylic group in aromatic ring besides amino group in aromatic ring.

Example: Isomeric nitro aniline, sulphanilic acid and anthranilic acid.

Fast diazotisable compounds do not contain any substituent group other than amino group but sometimes they may contain $-CH_3$ or $-OH$ group along with NH_2 group.

Example: aniline, toluidine and aminophenol.

Adding KBr to the solution can increase the rate of titration. In case of slowly diazotisable compound sufficient time (5–10 min) should be given to the solution under test. So that last portion of nitrous acid could fully react with amine.

If the test for endpoint determination is carried out immediately after addition of the sodium nitrite, the nitrous acid so formed, which has not yet entered into the reaction with amine, will be taken as excess nitrous acid, indicating the endpoint has reached. By sufficient stirring and slow addition of $NaNO_2$ and keeping in view the time factor, a large excess of $NaNO_2$ is not allowed to build up. It is also suggested that the burette tip is placed below the surface of reaction mixture to prevent the loss of HNO_2.

(2) **Temperature:** The diazonium compounds so formed are unstable and readily decompose at elevated temperature. This can lead to side reaction and give wrong result. To eliminate this, titration is carried out at low temperature (0–10°C), optimum temperature for most amine is 10–15°C, when they form relatively stable diazo compounds.

EXPERIMENT 39

Assay of calcium aminosalicylate content in tablets

Calcium aminosalicylate, $2(C_7H_6NO_3).Ca.3H_2O$ is a salt of 4-aminosalicylic acid, used for the treatment of tuberculosis.

Experimental overview

The reaction of calcium aminosalicylate with sodium nitrite forms a diazonium salt.

Calcium aminosalicylate   Diazotised calcium aminosalicylate

The presence of a small excess of nitrous acid indicates the endpoint which is detected using starch–iodide paper as an external indicator.

$$KI + HCl \longrightarrow HI + KCl$$

$$2HI + 2HNO_2 \longrightarrow I_2 + 2NO + 2H_2O$$

The liberated iodine reacts with starch to impart a blue color. The endpoint may also be detected electrometrically.

Reagents required

1. Standard 0.1 M $NaNO_2$ solution. Dissolve 7.5 g sodium nitrite in sufficient water to make 1000 ml.
2. Hydrochloric acid.
3. Starch iodide paper.

Procedure

1. **Standardization of 0.1 M $NaNO_2$ solution:** For standardization, dissolve an accurately weighed sample of sulfanilamide (about 1 g), previously dried at 105°C for 2 hrs, in concentrated hydrochloric acid (40 ml) and water (100 ml). Cool the solution to about 5°C and titrate with 0.1 M sodium nitrate dipping the tip of burette well in the solution. Add sodium nitrite slowly until an immediate blue color is obtained on placing a drop of the solution to a starch–iodide paper. The endpoint should be reproducible for a period of at least 1 minute.

   Nitrous acid is formed from sodium nitrite in acidic medium which diazotizes sulphanilamide to form the diazonium salt.

$$NaNO_2 + HCl \longrightarrow HNO_2 + NaCl$$

$$H_2NSO_2-C_6H_4-NH_2 + HNO_2 + HCl \longrightarrow H_2NSO_2-C_6H_4-N_2Cl + 2H_2O$$

Sulfanilamide $\qquad\qquad\qquad\qquad\qquad$ Diazotised sulfanilamide

At the endpoint, a slight excess of nitrous acid reacts with starch iodide paper to give the blue color.

Each ml of 0.1 M $NaNO_2$ solution = 0.01732 g of sulphanilamide.

2. **Determination of calcium aminosalicylate tablet:**
   (i) Weigh and powder 20 tablets. Find out the average weight of tablet.
   (ii) Weigh accurately powder equivalent to 0.4 g of calcium amino salicylate and dissolve in 25 ml of water and shake frequently for 10 minutes or until all the calcium aminosalicylate dissolves.
   (iii) Add 10 ml of hydrochloric acid, 1 g of potassium bromide and 50 ml of water.
   (iv) Cool to below 15°C and slowly titrate with 0.1 M sodium nitrite at a temperature until a drop of the solution immediately gives a blue color when drawn quickly by means of a fine rod across the surface of a starch iodide paper. The titration is completed when the endpoint is reproducible after the titrated solution has been allowed to stand for 5 minutes. The endpoint may be determined by electrometric method.

   Note: Keep the tip of burette well below the surface of liquid.

Observation and calculation

Weight of tablet powder = W g

Average weight of tablet = Y g

Volume of 0.1 M $NaNO_2$ consumed = V ml

From the reaction:

Molecular weight of calcium aminosalicylate = 344.34

2 moles of 1 M $NaNO_2$ = 1 mole of calcium aminosalicylate ($C_{14}H_{12}CaN_2O_6.3H_2O$)

1 ml of 0.1 M $NaNO_2$ solution = 0.01722 g of $C_{14}H_{12}CaN_2O_6.3H_2O$

V ml of 0.1M $NaNO_2$ solution = 0.01722 × V g of $C_{14}H_{12}CaN_2O_6.3H_2O$

W g of powder contain = 0.01722 × V g of $C_{14}H_{12}CaN_2O_6.3H_2O$

The content of calcium aminosalicylate in tablet

$$= \frac{0.01722 \times V \times \text{Molarity (cal.)}}{\text{Molarity (given)} \times W} \times Y = ... \text{ g of } C_{14}H_{12}CaN_2O_6.3H_2O$$

% content of calcium aminosalicylate = $\dfrac{\text{Practical value}}{\text{Theoretical value}} \times 100 = ...\%$

Result: The % content of calcium aminosalicylate in tablet is found to be ... .

Judge yourself

1. Why tip of burette is kept well below the surface of liquid during the titration?
2. Why KBr is added in diazotization method?
3. Why titration is performed slowly?
4. How chloramphenicol and succinyl sulfathiazole are assayed by diazotisation method?

EXPERIMENT 40

Determination of sulfamethoxazole content in co-trimoxazole tablets

Co-trimoxazole tablet is a combination of trimethoprim (80 mg to 160 mg) and sulphamethoxazole (400 mg to 800 mg) and results in synergistic bactericidal effects. The action of co-trimoxazole is achieved by the sequential blocking of two enzymes essential in folinic acid synthesis in the organism. Sulfamethoxazole inhibits bacterial synthesis of dihydrofolic acid by competing with PABA. Trimethoprim blocks production of tetrahydrofolic acid by inhibiting the enzyme dihydrofolate reductase. This combination blocks 2 consecutive steps in bacterial biosynthesis of essential nucleic acids and proteins and is usually bactericidal.

Experimental overview

Sulfamethoxazole is determined by diazotization method due to presence of primary aromatic amino group.

Sulfamethoxazole   Diazotized sulfamethoxazole

When sulfmethoxazole is completely diazotized by nitrous acid (liberated from the reaction of $NaNO_2$ and HCl), a slight excess of nitrous acid reacts with starch–iodide paper to mark the endpoint (blue color).

$$2KI + 2HNO_2 + 2HCl \longrightarrow 2KCl + I_2 + 2NO + 2H_2O$$

$$I_2 + Starch \longrightarrow Blue \ color \ (endpoint)$$

Reagent required

1. Standard 0.1 M $NaNO_2$ solution. Dissolve 7.5 g sodium nitrite in sufficient water to make 1000 ml.
2. Hydrochloric acid
3. Starch–iodide paper

Procedure

1. **Standardization of 0.1 M $NaNO_2$ solution:** For standardization, dissolve an accurately weighed sample of sulfanilamide (about 1 g), previously dried at 105°C for 2 hrs, in concentrated hydrochloric acid (40 ml) and water (100 ml). Cool the solution to about 5°C and titrate with 0.1 M sodium nitrate dipping the tip of burette well in the solution. Add sodium nitrite slowly until an immediate blue color is obtained on placing a drop of the solution to a starch–iodide paper. The endpoint should be reproducible for a period of at least 1 minute.

   Nitrous acid is formed from sodium nitrite in acidic medium which diazotizes sulphanilamide to form the diazonium salt.

$$NaNO_2 + HCl \longrightarrow HNO_2 + NaCl$$

$$H_2NSO_2-C_6H_4-NH_2 + HNO_2 + HCl \longrightarrow H_2NSO_2-C_6H_4-N_2Cl + 2H_2O$$

Sulfanilamide   Diazotised sulfanilamide

At the endpoint, a slight excess of nitrous acid reacts with starch–iodide paper to give the blue color.

Each ml of 0.1 M NaNO$_2$ solution = 0.01722 g of sulphanilamide.

2. **Determination of sulfamethoxazole:**
   (i) Weigh and powder 20 tablets. Determine average weight of the tablet.
   (ii) Dissolve a quantity of the powder equivalent to 0.5 g of sulfamethoxazole in 60 ml of water and 10 ml of HCl solution.
   (iii) Cool down the mixture below 10°C and titrate slowly with 0.1 M NaNO$_2$ solution until a drop of reaction mixture gives immediate blue color with starch iodide paper (endpoint). Note down the titre value 'V' ml.

   Note: The endpoint can also be determined potentiomerically.

Observation and calculation

Average weight of tablet: Y g

Weight of powder: W g

Amount of 0.1 M NaNO$_2$ consumed: V ml

Molecular weight of sulfamethoxazole = 253.3

According to above reaction:

i mole of sulfamethoxazole (C$_{10}$H$_{11}$N$_3$O$_3$S) = 1 mole of 1 M NaNO$_2$ = 1/10 of 0.1 M NaNO$_2$

Hence, 1 ml of 0.1 M NaNO$_2$ solution = 0.02533 g of C$_{10}$H$_{11}$N$_3$O$_3$S

V ml of 0.1 M NaNO$_2$ solution = 0.02533 × V g of C$_{10}$H$_{11}$N$_3$O$_3$S

The content of sulfamethoxazole in W g of powder = 0.02453 × V g of C$_{10}$H$_{11}$N$_3$O$_3$S

The content of sulfamethoxazole in tablet

$$= \frac{0.02533 \times V \times \text{Molarity (cal.)}}{\text{Molarity (given)} \times W} \times Y = ... \text{ g of } C_{10}H_{11}N_3O_3S$$

$$\% \text{ content of sulfamethoxazole} = \frac{\text{Practical value}}{\text{Theoretical value}} \times 100 = ...\%$$

Result

The % content of sulfamethoxazole is found to be … .

Judge yourself

1. How sulfamethoxazole and trimethoprim show synergistic action? Explain.
2. How the endpoint in diazotization titration is detected?
3. Why tip of burette is immersed in sulfa drug solution in nitrite titration?
4. Why NaNO$_2$ solution is standardized?

EXPERIMENT 41

Determination of dapsone content in dapsone tablet

Dapsone (4,4′-diaminodiphenylsulfone, DDS) is a primary treatment for **dermatitis herpetiformis.** It is an antibacterial drug for susceptible cases of leprosy. It is a white, odorless crystalline powder, practically insoluble in water and insoluble in fixed and vegetable oils. Dapsone is issued on prescription in tablets of 25 and 100 mg. for oral use.

Experimental overview

Dapsone contains not less than 98.0% and not more than 102.0% of $C_{12}H_{12}N_2O_2S$, calculated on the dried basis.

Dapsone is determined by diazotization method due to presence of primary aromatic amino group.

When dapsone is completely diazotized by nitrous acid (liberated from the reaction of $NaNO_2$ and HCl), a slight excess of nitrous acid reacts with starch–iodide paper to mark the endpoint (blue color).

$$2KI + 2HNO_2 + 2HCl \longrightarrow 2KCl + I_2 + 2NO + 2H_2O$$

$$I_2 + Starch \longrightarrow Blue\ color\ (endpoint)$$

Reagents required

1. Standard 0.1 M $NaNO_2$ solution. Dissolve 7.5 g sodium nitrite in sufficient water to make 1000 ml.
2. Hydrochloric acid.
3. Starch iodide paper.

Procedure

Weigh 20 tablets and powder them. Weigh accurately powder equivalent to 0.25 g of dapsone and dissolve in 20 ml of water and 20 ml of hydrochloric acid. Cool the solution below 10°C temperature and titrate slowly with 0.1 M $NaNO_2$ solution until a drop of reaction mixture gives immediate blue color with starch–iodide paper (endpoint). Note down the titre value 'V' ml. Perform a blank titration.

Note: The endpoint can also be determined potentiomerically.

Observation and calculation

Average weight of tablet: Y g

Weight of powder: W g

Amount of 0.1 M $NaNO_2$ consumed by tablet powder : V_1 ml

Amount of 0.1 M $NaNO_2$ consumed in blank titration : V_2 ml

Difference: $V_1 - V_2 = V$ ml

According to above reaction:

Molecular weight of dapsone = 248.4

1 mole of dapsone $(C_{12}H_{12}N_2O_2S)$ = 2 moles of 1 M $NaNO_2$ = 2000 ml of 1 M $NaNO_2$

Hence, 1 ml of 0.1 M $NaNO_2$ solution = 0.01242 g of $C_{12}H_{12}N_2O_2S$

V ml of 0.1 M $NaNO_2$ solution = 0.01242 × V g of $C_{12}H_{12}N_2O_2S$

The content of dapsone in W g of powder = 0.01242 × V g of $C_{12}H_{12}N_2O_2S$

$$\text{The content of dapsone in tablet} = \frac{0.01242 \times V \times \text{Molarity (cal.)}}{\text{Molarity (given)} \times W} \times Y = ... \text{ g of } C_{12}H_{12}N_2O_2S$$

$$\% \text{ content of dapsone} = \frac{\text{Practical value}}{\text{Theoretical value}} \times 100 = ...\%$$

Result

The % content of dapsone is found to be ... .

Judge yourself

1. How the dapsone acts? Explain.
2. How the endpoint in diazotization titration is detected?
3. Give the reaction of dapsone with sodium nitrite.
4. Why nitrite titration is carried out at low temperature?

Kjeldahl Method

Introduction to Kjeldahl method

The Kjeldahl method was developed on 7th March 1883 for determining the nitrogen contents in organic and inorganic substances. Although the technique and apparatus have been modified over the years, the basic principles introduced by Johan Kjeldahl still endure today.

Kjeldahl nitrogen determinations are performed on a variety of substances such as meat, feed, grain, waste water, soil, and many other samples. The Kjeldahl method may be broken down into three main steps: digestion, distillation, and titration.

Digestion

Digestion is accomplished by boiling a homogeneous sample in concentrated sulfuric acid. The end result is an ammonium sulfate solution. The general equation for the digestion of an organic sample is shown below:

Organic (N) + H_2SO_4 → $(NH_4)_2SO_4$ + H_2O + CO_2 + other sample matrix byproducts

Distillation

Excess base is added to the digestion product to convert NH_4^+ ion to NH_3 as indicated in the following equation. The NH_3 is recovered by distilling the reaction product.

$$(NH_4)_2SO_4 + 2NaOH \xrightarrow{\text{Heat}} 2NH_3\uparrow + Na_2SO_4 + 2H_2O$$

Ammonium sulfate   **Ammonia gas**

Titration

Titration quantifies the amount of ammonia in the receiving solution. The amount of nitrogen in a sample can be calculated from the quantified amount of ammonia ion in the receiving solution.

There are two types of titration—back titration and direct titration. Both methods indicate the ammonia present in the distillate with a color change.

In back titration (commonly used in macro Kjeldahl), the ammonia gas is captured by a carefully measured excess of a standardized acid solution in the receiving flask. The excess of acid in the receiving solution keeps the pH low, and the indicator does not change until the solution is "back titrated" with base.

$$2NH_3 + 2H_2SO_4 \longrightarrow (NH_4)_2SO_4 + H_2SO_4$$

| Ammonia | Standard sulfuric acid | Ammonium sulfate | Sulfuric acid |

(no color change)

$$(NH_4)_2SO_4 + H_2SO_4 + 2NaOH \longrightarrow Na_2SO_4 + (NH_4)_2SO_4 + 2H_2O$$

| Ammonia sulfate | Measured excess | Measured sodium hydroxide | Ammonium sulfate |

(color change occurs)

In direct titration, if boric acid is used as the receiving solution instead of a standardized mineral acid, the chemical reaction is:

$$NH_3 + H_3BO_3 \longrightarrow NH_4^+H_2BO_3^- + H_3BO_3$$

| Ammonia gas | Boric acid | Ammonium-borate complex | Excess boric acid |

(color change occurs)

The boric acid captures the ammonia gas, forming an ammonium–borate complex. As the ammonia collects, the color of the receiving solutions changes in presence of acid. Mixtures of methyl red and tetrabromophenol or methyl red and methylene blue (2:1) or methyl red alone were suggested as indicators.

$$2NH_4^+H_2BO_3^- + H_2SO_4 \longrightarrow (NH_4)_2SO_4 + 2H_3BO_3$$

| Ammonium-borate complex | | Boric acid |

(color change occurs in reverse)

The boric acid method has the advantages that only one standard solution is necessary for the determination and that the solution has a long shelf life.

EXPERIMENT 42

Determination of nitrogen/protein content

Experimental overview

The **Kjeldahl method** in analytical chemistry is a method for the quantitative determination of nitrogen in chemical substances developed by **Johan Kjeldahl**. The method consists of heating a substance with sulfuric acid which decomposes the organic nitrogen present to ammonium sulfate. In this step, potassium sulfate is added in order to increase the boiling point of the medium (from 337 to 373°C). Chemical decomposition of the sample is complete when the medium has become clear and colorless (initially very dark). Potassium sulfate (K_2SO_4) (also known as potash of sulfur) is a non-flammable white crystalline salt which is soluble in water.

The solution is then distilled with sodium hydroxide (added in small quantities) which converts the ammonium salt to ammonia. The amount of ammonia present (hence the amount of nitrogen present in the sample) is determined by back titration. The end of the condenser is dipped into a solution of hydrochloric acid or sulfuric acid of precisely known concentration. The ammonia reacts with the acid and the remainder of the acid is then titrated with a standard sodium hydroxide solution with a phenolphthalein pH indicator.

$$Protein + H_2SO_4 \longrightarrow CO_2 + (NH_4)_2SO_4 + SO_2$$
$$(NH_4)_2SO_4 + 2NaOH \longrightarrow Na_2SO_4 + NH_4OH$$
$$2NH_4OH + H_2SO_4 \longrightarrow (NH_4)_2SO_4 + 2H_2O$$

Now-a-days, the Kjeldahl method is largely automated and makes use of specific catalysts (mercury oxide or copper sulfate) to speed up the decomposition. The Kjeldahl method's universality, precision and reproducibility have made it the internationally-recognized method for estimating the protein content in foods and it is the standard method against which all other methods are judged. It does not, however, give a measure of true protein content, as it measures non-protein nitrogen in addition to the nitrogen in proteins. Also, different correction factors are needed for different proteins to account for different amino acid sequences.

Reagents required

1. Sulfuric acid, concentrated, 95–98%, reagent grade.
2. 0.1 N sodium hydroxide solution.
3. Potassium sulfate (K_2SO_4).
4. Anhydrous copper sulfate ($CuSO_4$).
5. 0.5 N hydrochloric acid. Prepare by diluting 43.0 ml 36.5 to 38% HCl to 1.0 litre with distilled water.

Procedure

The procedure in Kjeldahl method consists of three steps:

A. Digestion

1. Weigh approximately 1 g powdered sample into digestion flask, recording weight (*W*) to nearest 0.1 mg. Include reagent blank and high purity lysine HCl as check of correctness of digestion parameters.
2. Add 15 g potassium sulfate, 0.04 g anhydrous copper sulfate, 0.5 to 1.0 g alundum granules, or add 16.7 g K_2SO_4, 0.01 g anhydrous copper sulfate, 0.6 g TiO_2 and 0.3 g pumice. Then,

add 20 ml sulfuric acid (add additional 1.0 ml sulfuric acid for each 0.1 g fat or 0.2 g other organic matter if sample weight is greater than 1 g).

3. Heat samples on the digestion unit (heater setting 5–7) while aspirating.
4. With a hot glove or tongs, rotate flasks occasionally to prevent sticking and to expose all surfaces to acid.
5. Heat until samples are clear (this may take 30–45 minutes). *Some samples will be clear with a slight color pigment.*
6. When complete, cool flasks for 5 to 10 minutes.
7. Add 10 ml of distilled water to the cooled digestion flask for transferring to the distillation unit.

B. Distillation

Distillation consists of addition of excess base to the acid digested mixture to convert ammonium ion to NH_3 gas, followed by boiling and condensation of NH_3 gas in a receiving solution.

1. Prepare titration flask by adding appropriate volume of accurately measured standard HCl solution to amount of water so that condenser tip is immersed (try 15 ml acid and 70 ml water if undecided). For reagent blank, pipet 1 ml of acid and add approximately 85 ml water. Add 3 to 4 drops methyl red indicator solution.
2. Add 2 to 3 drops of tributyl citrate or other antifoam agent to digestion flask to reduce foaming.
3. Slowly transfer the content to distillation flask, add sufficient 45% sodium hydroxide solution (approximately 80 ml) to make mixture strongly alkali (do not mix until after flask is connected to distillation apparatus otherwise ammonia will be lost).
4. Heat to distill out the ammonia which is collected in titration flask containing hydrochloric acid.
5. Remove the titration flask from unit, rinsing the condenser tube with distilled water as the flask is being removed.

C. Titration

There are two types of titration—back titration and direct titration. Both the methods indicate the ammonia present in the distillate with a color change and allow for calculation of unknown concentration. Titrate excess acid with standard sodium hydroxide solution to orange endpoint (color change from red to orange to yellow) and record volume to nearest 0.01 ml Titrate the reagent blank similarly.

Comments

- Reagent proportions, heat input and digestion time are critical factors for good result.
- Ratio of salt to acid (wt:vol) should be 1:1 at end of digestion for proper temperature control. Digestion may be incomplete at lower ratio; nitrogen may be lost at higher ratio. Each gram of fat consumes 10 ml sulfuric acid and each gram of carbohydrate consumes 4 ml sulfuric acid during digestion.

Observation and calculation

The calculation can either be performed as percent nitrogen or percent protein.

For percent nitrogen:

Let, mass of the organic compound = W g

Vol. of the std. acid required for complete neutralization of the evolved ammonia = V ml

Normality of the standard HCl = N

From the law of equivalence (normality equation),

1000 ml of 1 N HCl = 1000 ml of 1 N NH_3 = 17 g NH_3 = 14 g nitrogen

Then, V ml of N acid = V ml of NH_3

NV milliequivalent of acid = NV milliequivalent of ammonia

Therefore, mass of nitrogen in the evolved ammonia = $\dfrac{14 \times N \times V}{1000}$ g

Then, percentage of nitrogen in the sample = $\dfrac{14NV}{1000} \times \dfrac{100}{W} = \dfrac{1.4\ NV}{W}$

It has been shown that protein contains 16% nitrogen. (wheat and dairy products are some exceptions.) By dividing 100 by 16, we get the conversion factor for nitrogen to protein of 6.25. Hence, the percent protein is calculated as follows:

$$\% \text{ Protein} = 6.25 \times \% \text{ N}$$

Following is a list of acceptable standards available to include in Kjeldahl runs.

Theoretical yield standard	% nitrogen
Ammonium p-toluenesulfonate	7.402
Glycine p-toluenesulfonate	5.665
Nicotinic acid p-toluenesulfonate	4.743
Lysine monohydrochloride	15.34
Ammonium chloride (100% assay)	26.18
Ammonium sulfate (100% assay)	21.20
Ammonium dihydrogen phosphate	12.15
Urea	46.63

The ammonium salts and glycine p-toluenesulfonate serve primarily as a check on distillation efficiency and accuracy in titration steps because they are digested very readily. Lysine and nicotinic acid are difficult to digest, therefore serve as a check on digestion efficiency.

Sample calculation

The ammonia evolved from 0.21 g of an organic compound by Kjeldahl method neutralised 15 ml of N/20 sulfuric acid solution. Calculate the percentage of nitrogen.

Weight of organic compound = 0.21 g

Normality of acid = $N/20$

Volume of standard acid neutralised by ammonia = 15 ml

1000 ml of 1 N ammonia contains = 14 g of nitrogen

15 ml of ammonia of normality $\dfrac{N}{20}$ contains nitrogen $= \dfrac{14 \times 15 \times 1}{1000 \times 20}$

0.21 g of compound contains nitrogen $= \dfrac{14 \times 15}{1000 \times 20}$

100 g of compound contains nitrogen $= \dfrac{14 \times 15 \times 100}{1000 \times 20 \times 0.21} = 5$ g

∴ percentage of nitrogen = 5.

Result

The % protein content present in the sample is found to be ... %.

Judge yourself

1. What is the advantage of using boric acid to detect the endpoint?
2. Why digestion of sample is carried out in Kjeldahl method?
3. How % nitrogen content is related to protein content in the sample?
4. Write down the purpose of distillation and explain each step in the digestion by writing chemical reactions.

Karl Fischer Titration

Introduction

Karl Fischer titration is the most important volumetric method of water (moisture) determination. It determines the water content in liquid and solid materials with the involvement of Karl Fischer reagent.

Karl Fischer reagent

Traditionally, Karl Fischer reagent (KF) is a solution of iodine and sulphur dioxide in methanol and pyridine. Traditional KF reagent is slow in reactivity and has unpleasant odour. Newly developed pyridine-free KF reagents substitute various proprietary amines for pyridine. Methanol is replaced by 2-methoxy ethanol or xylene. If methanol is incompatible with the sample (like aldehydes or ketones), the Hydra-point solvent K_1 or K_2 can be used to dissolve the sample.

Replacement of components like pyridine and methanol with other amines and 2-methoxy ethanol respectively increases the speed as well as removes the foul smell of pyridine.

Basic principle

The method depends upon the reaction of water which is being determined, with iodine and sulfur dioxide in pyridine–methanol system as follows:

$$I_2 + SO_2 + H_2O \longrightarrow 2HI + SO_3 \qquad \text{... (1)}$$

$$\underset{\text{Pyridine}}{C_5H_5N} + SO_3 \longrightarrow \underset{\text{Pyridine-sulfur trioxide}}{C_5H_5N.SO_3} \qquad \text{... (2)}$$

$$C_5H_5N.SO_3 + CH_3OH \longrightarrow C_5H_5NH^+CH_3-O-SO_3^- \qquad \text{... (3)}$$

$$2HI + 2C_5H_5N \longrightarrow 2C_5H_5NH + I^- \qquad \text{... (4)}$$

The above equations, 1 to 4, indicate that 1 mole of water is equivalent to 1 mole of I_2. The reoxidation of HI formed in reaction (Eq. 1) is prevented by formation of complex between pyridine and sulfur trioxide (Eq. 4). The reverse reaction may take place if the concentration of acidic products, SO_3 and HI, becomes high.

The complex of pyridine with sulfur trioxide may further react with another water molecule if methanol is not present in the system.

$$C_5H_5N.SO_3 + H_2O \longrightarrow C_5H_5NH^+HSO_4^-$$

Hence, KF reagent consists of iodine, sulfur trioxide, pyridine and methanol.

Pyridine performs two functions:

  (i) It prevents the loss of SO_3 from KF reagent by forming an addition compound.

  (ii) It assists in completion of reaction of I_2 and SO_3 with water by combining the products of the reaction as shown by 2 and 4.

For every mole of iodine in the reagent, it is necessary that 3 moles of pyridine and 1 mole of SO_3 must be present otherwise the color of iodine will not be destroyed.

In conclusion, basic equation (1) of Karl Fischer titration indicates that in presence of water, iodine passes into the combined state. From the volume of SO_2 and I_2 consumed, quantity of water can be calculated. An endpoint is determined visually from the presence of excess of iodine or using endpoint sensing electrode on autotitrator.

Hydra-point Karl Fischer reagents

These are available in one and two component systems.

One component system is meant for high volume use. In this, all the reactants (I_2 and SO_2) are present in one system. The sample is dissolved in methanol in titration flask and composite reagent is added until the endpoint is obtained (presence of little excess of iodine). In this system, there is side reaction and hence, the reagent deteriorates on standing and loses half its strength within a month.

$$I_2 + SO_3 + 3C_5H_5N + CH_3OH \longrightarrow C_5H_5NCH_3{}^+ CH_3SO_4^- + 2C_5H_5NH^+I^-$$

For this reason, *two component system is used* in which the titrant has the I_2 constituent and the solvent has the SO_2 constituent. The Karl Fischer reaction completes when both the components are present together. Therefore, Hydra-point two component system is extremely stable.

Method (volumetric)

Fill the burette with titrant (one component reagent) and add 20–30 ml of anhydrous methanol to the titration vessel. Titrate the methanol in the titration vessel to dryness. Add accurately weighed amount of sample (of which water content is to be determined) to the titration vessel and titrate the sample in the titration vessel to dryness. Based on the titre and the volume of titrant consumed, calculate the water content.

Preparation of Karl Fischer reagent

Mix in a combustion flask 400 ml of dehydrated methanol and 80 g of dehydrated pyridine. Immerse the flask in ice and bubble the dried SO_2 slowly through the mixture until its weight increases by 20 g. Add 45 g of I_2 and shake well until it dissolves. Keep the solution for 24 hours before use; this solution deteriorates gradually, therefore it should be standardized within one hour before use.

Standardization of KF reagent

The KF reagent requires standardization before use. This can be done by using either standard solution of water in methanol or hydrated salt like sodium tartrate ($Na_2C_4H_4O_6.2H_2O$). Take accurately weighed quantity (0.5–0.7 g sodium tartrate) in 40 ml of dry methanol and titrate with KF reagent till endpoint. The KF reagent on reaction with content gives lemon yellow color and at the endpoint, color changes due to presence of excess of iodine.

Each mg of sodium tartrate = 2 moles of water = 36 g of water.

To eliminate interference from atmospheric moisture, the titration should be carried out under an atmosphere of dry nitrogen.

Caulometric Karl Fischer titrations

Caulometric titrations are specially well suited for samples with low water content (0.1–0.0001%) or colored sample. The caulometric titrations use the same reaction mechanism as KF volumetric method.

$$H_2O + SO_2 + I_2 \longrightarrow 2HI + SO_3$$

The difference lies in the source of iodine. In volumetric method, the iodine is introduced from the reagent while in caulometric titrations, the iodine is electrochemically generated from the oxidation of an iodide. The iodine is then consumed in KF reaction.

$$2I^- \longrightarrow I_2$$

The iodine continues to be generated by the titrator until an endpoint is obtained. The titrator calculates the amount of iodine generated based on the amount of current needed to reach an endpoint.

EXPERIMENT 43

Determination of moisture content in amoxycillin trihydrate

Amoxycillin trihydrate, $C_{16}H_{19}N_3O_5.3H_2O$ is white to off white crystalline powder. It is a broad-spectrum β-lactam antibiotic.

Amoxycillin trihydrate

Experimental view

A dehydrating solvent suitable for the sample is placed in a flask. Titrant is used to remove all moisture from the solvent. The sample is then added. Titration is carried out using a titrant, the titre (mg H_2O/ml) of which has previously been determined. The moisture content of the sample is determined from the titration volume (ml). The endpoint is detected using the constant-current polarization voltage method.

Also see the introduction part.

Amoxycillin trihydrate IP contains 11.5–14.5% w/w of moisture content.

Procedure

1. **Standardization of Karl Fischer reagent:** Accurately weigh about 50 mg of water and titrate with Karl Fischer reagent till the endpoint. Note the titre value (V_1 ml). Alternatively, it can be standardized with the help of sodium tartrate as mention in introduction part of this chapter.
2. Transfer sufficient dried methanol in a titration vessel and titrate with Karl Fischer reagent till the endpoint (**Note:** It is done to eliminate the possible moisture present in methanol).
3. Accurately weigh about 0.6 g of amoxicillin trihydrate and dissolve into the above methanol with stirring. Titrate with Karl Fischer reagent till the endpoint. Note the titre value (V_2 ml).

Observation and calculation

Weight of water: W g

Weight of amoxicillin trihydrate: W_1 g

Volume of KF reagent required to titrate water for standardization: V_1 ml

Volume of KF reagent required to titrate amoxicillin trihydrate: V_2 ml

$$\text{The percentage of moisture content} = \frac{W \times V_2}{V_1 \times W_1} \times 100 = \dots. \text{ moisture content}$$

Result

The % moisture content of amoxicillin trihydrate: ....% w/w.

Judge yourself

1. What are the applications of Karl Fischer methods?
2. Name the other methods which are used to determine the moisture.
3. What is the role of pyridine in Karl Fischer titration?
4. Name the amine which can substitute the pyridine in KF reagent.

Polarimetry

Introduction

Polarimetry is commonly used to analyze chiral substances. Most of the biomolecules are chiral and hence, rotate polarized light. Carbohydrates are particularly amenable for analysis using polarimetry. The magnitude and direction of rotation of the plane of polarized light by an asymmetric compound is a specific physical property of the compound that may be used for its characterization. When plane polarized light is passed through a solution of a pure asymmetric compound, the extent of rotation depends upon the concentration of the compound, the length of the light path through the solution, the wavelength of the light, and the temperature. These variables are related by the **Biot's** law:

$$[\alpha]_D^T = \frac{[\alpha]_{obs}}{l \times c}$$

where

$[\alpha]_D^T$ = specific rotation of the compound at temperature T using the D line of the sodium spectrum as the light source

$[\alpha]_{obs}$ = observed angle of rotation

l = path length through the solution in decimeters (usually 2 dm).

c = concentration of the compound in g/100 ml.

How to measure angle of rotation from polarimeter

Polarimeter (Fig. 9.1) consists of light source, a polarizer, an analyzer attached to disk graduated in degrees and fraction of degrees, sample tube and half shadow device.

Sodium vapor lamp is used as light source.

Two different nicol prisms are used as polarizer and analyser in most of the polarimeter. Monochromatic light is plane polarized by the stationary polarizer and extent of rotation of this polarized light is related to rotation of the analyzer. The no. of degrees of rotation of the analyzer is read on the graduated disk attached to it.

Polarimeter tubes are the container for the sample to be analysed and are placed between the polarizer and analyzer in the path of the plane polarised light.

Because it is easier for the human eye to match two adjacent areas to same degrees of brightness than to determine a point of maximum darkness or brightness, a third Nicol prism is placed behind

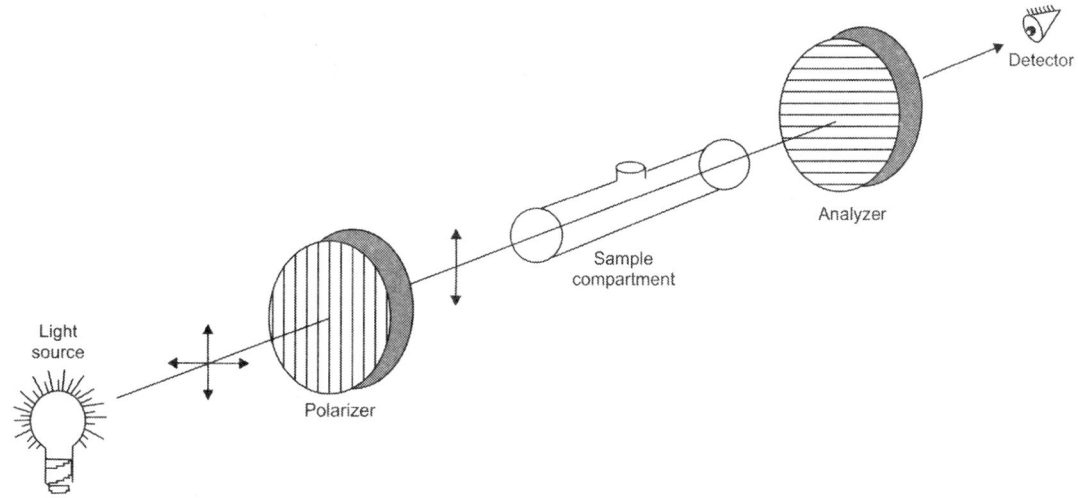

Fig. 9.1: Schematic representation of polarimeter.

the polarizer and rotated through a small angle to divide the field into halves of unequal brightness. An eyepiece is focused on the field and by rotating the analyzer, the two halves may be brought to equal brightness (Fig. 9.2). This is called balance or zero point.

When an optically active substance is placed in the path of plane polarized light, one half appears

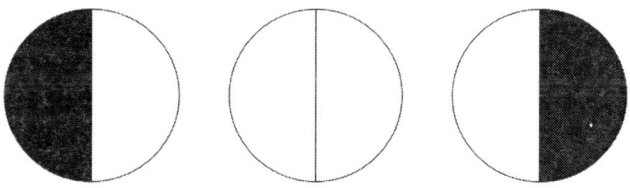

Fig. 9.2: Field view.

dark and other half appears bright. Rotation of analyzer returns the two halves to equal intensity of illumination. The number of degrees of rotation (either in left direction or right direction) as read on graduated disk measures the optical activity.

Applications

Polarimetry is helpful in determining product purity by measuring specific rotation and optical rotation of:

- Amino acids
- Steroids
- Tranquilizers
- Serums
- Antibiotics
- Amino sugars
- Analgesics
- Vitamins.
- Dextrose
- Cocaine
- Codeine

EXPERIMENT 44

Quantitative determination of sugar by polarimetric method

Experimental overview

Polarimetry is used in carbohydrate chemistry, especially in the analysis of sugar solutions. Polarimetry is a sensitive, non-destructive technique for measuring the optical activity exhibited by inorganic and organic compounds. The optically active molecule like sugar molecules rotate the polarised light when passing through it. The amount of optical rotation is determined by the molecular structure and concentration of chiral molecules in the substance. Each optically active substance has its own specific rotation as defined in Biot's law:

$$[\alpha]_D^T = \frac{[\alpha]_{obs}}{l \times c}$$

where

$[\alpha]_D^T$ = specific rotation of the compound at temperature T using the D line of the sodium spectrum as the light source

$[\alpha]_{obs}$ = observed angle of rotation

l = path length through the solution in decimeters (usually 2 dm).

c = concentration of the compound in g/100 ml.

For quantitative estimation, calibration curve is constructed by plotting a graph between specific rotation and sugar. From the calibration curve, the concentration of unknown sample is read out.

Reagents required

1. Dextrose (reference substance).
2. Water.

Procedure

(i) Prepare 5%, 10%, 15% dextrose solutions and measure the angle of rotation as mentioned in the introduction part..

(ii) Record in Table 9.1 as given below.

(iii) Similarly, measure the angle of rotation in unknown solution.

Observation and calculation

Table 9.1: Measurement of specific rotation

S. No.	% of dextrose	Angle of rotation
1	Distilled water	—
2	5%	—
3	10%	—
4	15%	—
5	Test solution	—

Calculate the specific rotation of each solution by the formula:

$$[\alpha]_D^T = \frac{[\alpha]_{obs}}{l \times c}$$

Plot a graph between specific rotation and concentration of dextrose solution and read out the concentration (%) of dextrose in test solution.

Alternate method

(i) Measure the angle of rotation/specific rotation of known standard, for example 10%.
(ii) Similarly, measure the angle of rotation/specific rotation of unknown solution.

Weight of known standard = W_1 g

Volume of water in which known standard is dissolved = V_1 ml

Volume of unknown sample = V_2 ml

Specific rotation of known standard = A

Specific rotation of unknown sample = B

Concentration of sucrose in unknown sample = W_2 (in question, which is dissolved in V_2 ml)

$$A \times \frac{W_1}{V_1} = B \times \frac{W_2}{V_2}$$

Concentration (W_2) of sucrose in unknown sample $= \dfrac{A \times W_1 \times V_2}{V_1 \times B}$

For determination of purity of sucrose:

$$\% \text{ purity} = \frac{B}{A} \times \frac{W_1}{V_1} \times \frac{V_2}{W_2} \times 100$$

Judge yourself

1. What is plane polarized light?
2. What is specific rotation? Mention the factors affecting specific rotation.
3. What will be angle of rotation of sucrose after treatment with HCl solution?
4. Tick mark the correct word in the undermentioned questions:

Questions

1. The function of the polariser in a polarimeter is to:
   (a) rotate normal light
   (b) produce normal light
   (c) rotate plane polarised light
   (d) produce plane polarised light
2. One enantiomer of a compound is found to give a reading of +13.5° when inserted into a polarimeter. What reading would you expect the same amount of the other enantiomer to produce in the polarimeter?
   (a) 0°
   (b) +13.5°
   (c) −13.5°
   (d) +27°

Flame Photometry

Introduction

Flame photometry (also called flame atomic emission spectrometry) is a branch of atomic spectroscopy in which the species examined in the spectrometer are in the form of atoms. The other two branches of atomic spectroscopy are atomic absorption spectrophotometry (AAS) and inductively coupled plasma-atomic emission spectrometry (ICP-AES, a relatively new and very expensive technique not used in standard experiments). In all cases, the atoms under investigation are excited by light. Absorption techniques measure the absorbance of light due to the electrons going to a higher energy level.

Emission techniques measure the intensity of light that is emitted as electrons return to the lower energy levels.

Flame photometry is suitable for qualitative and quantitative determination of several cations, especially for metals that are easily excited to higher energy levels at a relatively low flame temperature (mainly Na, K, Rb, Cs, Ca, Ba, Cu). This technique uses a flame that evaporates the solvent and also sublimates and atomizes the metal and then excites a valence electron to an upper energy state. Light is emitted at characteristic wavelengths for each metal as the electron returns to the ground state that makes qualitative determination possible. Flame photometers use optical filters to monitor for the selected emission wavelength produced by the analyte species. Comparison of emission intensities of unknowns to either that of standard solutions (plotting calibration curve), or to those of an internal standard (standard addition method), allows quantitative analysis of the analyte metal in the sample solution. The intensity of the light emitted could be described by the Scheibe-Lomakin equation:

$$I = k \cdot c^n$$

where:

c = the concentration of the element

k = constant of proportionality

$n \sim 1$ (at the linear part of the calibration curve)

Then,

$$I = k \times c$$

This indicates that intensity of light is directly related to concentration of the sample.

Because of the very narrow and characteristic emission lines from the gas-phase atoms in the flame plasma, the method is relatively free of interferences from other elements. Therefore the flame photometry (as with other atomic spectroscopy methods) is very sensitive; measuring concentration of ppm magnitude (part per million, e.g. mg kg^{-1}) usually does not cause any problem.

The optimal concentration range of the solutions for the measured metal ion is 10^{-3}–10^{-4} mol dm^{-3}.

The flame photometers are relatively simply instruments. There is no need for source of light, since it is the measured constituent of the sample that is emitting the light. The energy that is needed for the excitation is provided by the temperature of the flame (2000–3000°C), produced by the burning of acetylene or natural gas (or propane-butane gas) in the presence of air or oxygen. By the heat of the flame and the effect of the reducing gas (fuel), molecules and ions of the sample species are decomposed and reduced to give atoms, e.g. $Na^+ + e^- \rightarrow Na$. Atoms in the vapor state give line spectra (not band spectra, because there are no covalent bonds hence there are not any vibrational sub-levels to cause broadening).

The most sensitive parts of the instrument are the aspirator and the burner. The gases play an important role in the aspiration and while making the aerosol. The air sucks up the sample (according to Bernoulli's principle) and passes it into the aspirator, where the bigger drops condense and could be eliminated. The monochromator selects the suitable (characteristic) wavelength of the emitted light. The usual optical filters could be used. The emitted light reaches the detector. This is a photo-multiplier producing an electric signal proportional to the intensity of emitted light (Fig. 10.1).

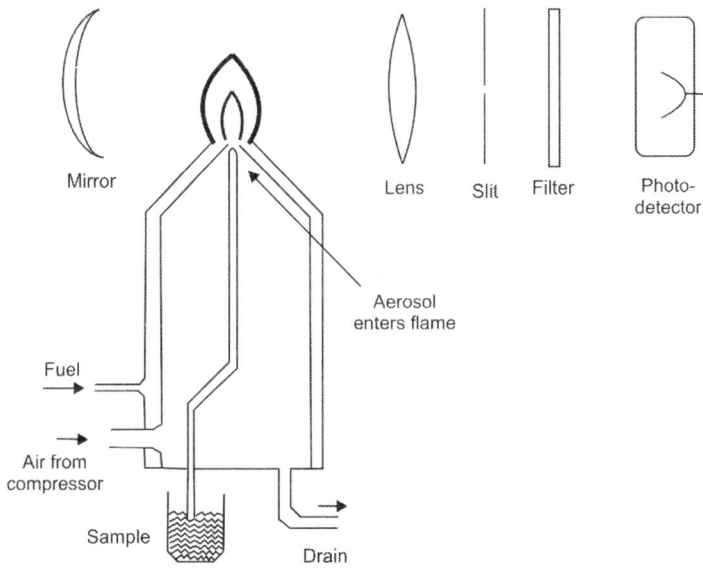

Fig. 10.1: Schematic diagram of flame photometer.

Flame photometry has many advantages. It is a simple, relatively inexpensive, high sample throughput method used for clinical, biological, and environmental analysis. On the other hand, the low temperature makes this method susceptible to, particularly, interference and the stability (or lack thereof) of the flame and aspiration conditions. Many different experimental variables affect the intensity of light emitted from the flame. Fuel and oxidant flow rates and purity, aspiration rates, solution viscosity, concomitants in the samples, etc. affect these.

Therefore, careful and frequent calibration is necessary for good results and it is very important to measure the emission from the standard and unknown solutions under conditions that are as nearly identical as possible.

EXPERIMENT 45

Determination of sodium and potassium ion concentrations in solution

Experimental overview

Flame photometry is a relatively old instrumental analysis method. Its origins date back to Bunsen's flame-color tests for the qualitative identification of select metallic elements. As an analytical method, atomic emission is a fast, simple, and sensitive method for the determination of trace metal ions in solution. Because of the very narrow (0.01 nm) and characteristic emission lines from the gas-phase atoms in the flame plasma, the method is relatively free of interferences from other elements.

The method is suitable for many metallic elements, especially for those metals that are easily excited to higher energy levels at the relatively cool temperatures of some flames—Li, Na, K, Rb, Cs, Ca, Cu, Sr, and Ba. Metalloids and nonmetals generally do not produce isolated neutral atoms in a flame, but mostly as polyatomic radicals and ions. Therefore, nonmetallic elements are not suitable for determination by flame emission spectroscopy, except for a very few and under very specialized conditions.

Reagents required

Standard sodium stock solution, 100.0 ppm

1. Accurately weigh out by difference 0.1271 g of reagent grade NaCl into a small weighing bottle. It is very difficult and time-consuming to weigh out exactly this amount. Get it as close as you reasonably can, record the exact mass, and correct your concentrations accordingly.

   Note : Mol. weight of NaCl = 58.5

   58.5 g NaCl/litre = 1000 ppm of NaCl

   58.5/23 g NaCl/litre = 1000 ppm for Na

   0.1271 g of NaCl/500 ml = 100 ppm of Na

2. Carefully transfer the salt quantitatively into a 500 ml volumetric flask. Use a few squirts of deionized water from your wash bottle on the weighing bottle and the sides of the flask to wash all of it down into the flask.

3. Add about 100 ml of deionized water to the flask, swirl several times, and dissolve all of the salt before diluting to volume with deionized water. This is critical.

Standard potassium stock solution, 100.0 ppm

Similarly, make the stock solution for potassium (atomic weight of K = 39 and Cl = 33.5).

Unknown solution

Obtain the unknown sample and carefully dilute to 100 ml mark with deionized water.

Procedure

Preparation of standard calibration solution: Pipet 10.00, 20.00, 30.00, 40.00, 50.00, 60.0, 70.0, 80.0, 90.0 ml of the standard 100 ppm sodium solution into different 100 ml volumetric flasks. This will give the concentration range of 10 to 90 ppm respectively. Dilute carefully to the mark with deionized water and mix thoroughly.

Instructions for use of the flame photometer

1. Ensure that the photometer drain is leading into a sink and that the instrument is connected to gas, air and electricity supplies. Ensure the mains supply gas tap is off.
2. Turn the "sensitivity" and instrument "gas" controls fully counterclockwise.
3. Insert the sodium optical filter (589 nm).
4. Switch on the instrument and unclamp the galvanometer by turning counterclockwise.
5. Open the mica window, turn on the mains gas supply, light the gas and close the window.
6. Turn on the air supply control and adjust the air pressure to 10 lb/in^2. Leave for 1–2 minutes to stabilize.
7. Place a beaker of distilled water into position at the left hand side of the instrument and insert the narrow draw tube into it to allow water to pass through the photometer.

    Note: once set up, the photometer must have water running through it at all times when a salt solution is not being measured. The rate of uptake is fast, so make sure there is always enough water in the beaker.
8. Adjust the gas control to give a flame with a large central blue cone. Then, with water passing through the instrument, slowly close the gas control until ten separate blue cones just form.
9. Set the galvanometer to zero using the "set zero" control.
10. Replace the distilled water with the NaCl solution (100 ppm standard) and adjust the "sensitivity" control till the galvanometer reads 100.
11. Quickly but carefully replace the NaCl standard with standards of decreasing concentration and note the readings in the table below.
12. Run water through the instrument again for 1–2 min, then place the draw tube into a beaker containing the unknown sachet solution and note the galvanometer reading.
13. Run water through the instrument again and replace the sodium with the potassium filter (766 nm).
14. Repeat the above procedure with the KCl standards, setting to 100 with most concentrated KCl standard, then reading the others in reverse order. Then, read the unknown solution.
16. Finally, run water through the instrument until the flame appears free of color again.
16. When the instrument is no longer required, switch off in the following sequence.
    (i)   Turn off the gas control and the mains gas supply.
    (ii) Wait for the flame to die out.
    (iii) Turn off the air supply.
    (iv) Switch off the electricity.
    (v)   Clamp the galvanometer.

Observation and calculation

Galvanometer reading

S. No.	Conc. of sodium (ppm)	Emission intensity	Conc. of potassium (ppm)	Emission intensity
1.	10	–	10	–
2.	20	–	20	–
3.	30	–	30	–
4.	40	–	40	–
5.	50	–	50	–
6.	60	–	60	–
7.	70	–	70	–
8.	80	–	80	–
9.	90	–	90	–
10.	100	–	100	–
11.	Unknown	–	Unknown	–

Plot a calibration curve by plotting the emission intensities as a function of Na concentration and potassium concentration separately. Determine the concentration of sodium and potassium unknown sample from the calibration curve.

Multiply with the dilution factor to get the concentration in original solution.

Result

The given solution contains sodium .... ppm and potassium .... ppm.

Judge yourself

1. Why deionised water is used?
2. Why the flame photometry is particularly useful for the determination of alkali and alkaline earth metal?
3. Mention the difference between flame photometry and atomic emission spectroscopy.
4. What is the importance of sodium and potassium ions in the body?
5. Which is the major extracellular cation present in the body?

EXPERIMENT 46

Determination of Na⁺ and K⁺ in oral rehydration sachet by flame photometry

Experimental overview

Potassium (K) is the major cation found inside of cells. The proper level of potassium is essential for normal cell function. An abnormal increase of potassium (hyperkalemia) or decrease of potassium (hypokalemia) can profoundly affect the nervous system and heart, and when extreme, can be fatal. The normal blood potassium level is 3.5–5.0 millimoles/liter (mmol/L).

Sodium (Na) is the major extracellular cation and it plays a role in body fluid distribution. Concentration of sodium ions inside the plasma (extracellular) is 130–145 mmol/L. Higher and lower concentrations are referred to as hypernatremia and hyponatremia, respectively.

When a solution containing cations of sodium and potassium is spayed into flame, the solvent evaporates and ions are converted into atomic state. In the heat of the flame (temperature about 1800°C), small fraction of the atoms is excited. Relaxation of the excited atoms to the lower energy level is accompanied by emission of light (photons) with characteristic wavelength (Na: 589 nm, K: 766 nm). Intensity of the emitted light depends on the concentration of particular atoms in flame.

Reagents required

Oral rehydration sachet:

NaCl standards: 0.25, 0.5, 1.0, 2.0, 4.0 and 5.0 mM (58.5/23 g of NaCl [in litre] = 1 mole of Na⁺).

KCl standards: 0.1, 0.2, 0.5, 1.0, 1.5, 2.0 mM (74.5/39 g KCl [in litre] = 1 mole of K⁺)

Procedure

1. Carefully open an oral rehydration sachet and empty the contents into a clean 250 ml beaker. Add about 150 ml distilled water and gently swirl the contents until dissolved.
2. Pour the solution into a 200 ml volumetric flask and rinse out the beaker with small amounts of distilled water, adding the washings to the flask. Finally, make up the flask to exactly 200 ml and mix thoroughly.
3. Make a 1/50 dilution of the redissolved sachet solution by accurately pipetting 2 ml of the solution into a 100 ml volumetric flask and making up to 100 ml with distilled water.

Instructions for use of the flame photometer

1. Ensure that the photometer drain is leading into a sink and that the instrument is connected to gas, air and electricity supplies. Ensure the mains supply gas tap is off.
2. Turn the "sensitivity" and instrument "gas" controls fully counterclockwise.
3. Insert the sodium optical filter (589 nm).
4. Switch on the instrument and unclamp the galvanometer by turning counterclockwise.
5. Open the mica window, turn on the mains gas supply, light the gas and close the window.
6. Turn on the air supply control and adjust the air pressure to 10 lb/in². Leave for 1–2 minutes to stabilise.

7. Place a beaker of distilled water into position at the left hand side of the instrument and insert the narrow draw tube into it to allow water to pass through the photometer.

   Note: once set up, the photometer must have water running through it at all times when a salt solution is not being measured. The rate of uptake is fast, so make sure there is always enough water in the beaker.

8. Adjust the gas control to give a flame with a large central blue cone then, with water passing through the instrument, slowly close the gas control until ten separate blue cones just form.

9. Set the galvanometer to zero using the "set zero" control.

10. Replace the distilled water with the 5 mM NaCl standard and adjust the "Sensitivity" control till the galvanometer reads 100.

11. Quickly but carefully, replace the 5 mM NaCl standard with standards of decreasing concentration from 4 mM to 0.25 mM and note the readings in the table below.

12. Run water through the instrument again for 1–2 min. Then place the draw tube into a beaker containing the 1 in 50 diluted rehydration sachet solution and note the galvanometer reading.

13. Run water through the instrument again and replace the sodium with the potassium filter (766 nm).

14. Repeat the above procedure with the KCl standards, setting to 100 with 2.0 mM KCl, then reading the others in reverse order. Then, read the 1 in 50 diluted rehydration sachet solution.

15. Finally, run water through the instrument until the flame appears free of color again.

16. When the instrument is no longer required, switch off in the following sequence.
   (i) Turn off the gas control and the mains gas supply.
   (ii) Wait for the flame to die out.
   (iii) Turn off the air supply.
   (iv) Switch off the electricity
   (v) Clamp the galvanometer.

Observation and calculation

Na^+ (mM)		5.0	4.0	2.0	1.0	0.5	0.25
Galvo reading	100°	–	–	–	–	–	–

K^+ (mM)		2.0	1.5	1.0	0.5	0.2	0.1
Galvo. reading	100°	–	–	–	–	–	–

Plot the galvanometer readings against Na^+ and K^+ concentrations on the graph paper provided (separate graph for each ion) and from these calibration curves determine the Na^+ and K^+ concentrations in the diluted sachet solution. Finally, calculate the Na^+ and K+ concentrations in the undiluted sachet solution.

Galvanometer Reading	Diluted concentration (mM)	Undiluted concentration (mM)
Sodium ion		
Potassium ion		

Result

Sodium ion ..... mM

Potassium ion ..... mM

Judge yourself

1. Explain the importance of sodium and potassium ions for human.
2. How the optical filter selects the particular wavelength?
3. What is composition of oral rehydration sachet?
4. How 0.25 mM solution of NaCl is prepared?

11

Fluorimetry

Introduction

Fluorometry or spectrofluorometry, is a type of electromagnetic spectroscopy which analyzes fluorescence from a sample. It involves using a beam of light, usually ultraviolet light, that excites the electrons in molecules of certain compounds and causes them to emit light of a lower energy, typically, but not necessarily, visible light. A complementary technique is absorption spectroscopy. Devices that measure fluorescence are called fluorometers or fluorimeters.

Molecules have various states referred to as energy levels. Fluorescence spectroscopy is primarily concerned with electronic and vibrational states. Generally, the species being examined will have a ground electronic state (a low energy state) of interest, and an excited electronic state of higher energy. Within each of these electronic states are various vibrational states.

In fluorescence spectroscopy, the species is first excited, by absorbing a photon, from its ground electronic state to one of the various vibrational states in the excited electronic state. Collisions with other molecules cause the excited molecule to lose vibrational energy until it reaches the lowest vibrational state of the excited electronic state.

The molecule then drops down to one of the various vibrational levels of the ground electronic state again, emitting a photon in the process. As molecules may drop down into any of several vibrational levels in the ground state, the emitted photons will have different energies, and thus frequencies. Therefore, by analysing the different frequencies of light emitted in fluorescent spectroscopy, along with their relative intensities, the structure of the different vibrational levels can be determined.

In a typical experiment, the different frequencies of fluorescent light emitted by a sample are measured, holding the excitation light at a constant wavelength. This is called an *emission spectrum*. An *excitation spectrum* is measured by recording a number of emission spectra using different wavelengths of excitation light.

EXPERIMENT 47

Fluorimetric determination of quinine

Quinine is an alkaloid occurring naturally in the bark of trees or shrubs of the various species of two Rubiaceous genera. The medicinal properties of Cinchona bark were first recognized in the seventeenth century and until 1942, quinine was the only existing specific antimalarial remedy. In recent years, however, another alkaloid quinidine, the stereoisomer of quinine has been used in the treatment of arrhythmia.

Experimental overview

Quinine shows the fluorescence which is the basis of its estimation. Molecular fluorescence occurs when a compound absorbs radiation, causing electrons to be promoted to excited states. As these excited states relax back to the ground state, light is emitted at wavelengths characteristic of the energy differences between the ground and excited states. At low concentrations the intensity of the fluorescence is proportional to concentration.

However, a variety of conditions adversely affect the linear relationship:

- Self quenching.
- External quenching.
- Decreased quantum efficiency.

Quinine

At high concentrations, however, the compound will absorb some of the fluoresced light, resulting in a non-linear dependence of the fluorescence intensity on the concentration.

Reagents required

1. Quinine sulfate.
2. Sulfuric acid.

Procedure

1. **Preparation of standard quinine sulfate solution:** Weigh accurately 10 mg of quinine sulfate, dissolve in sufficient quantity of 0.5 M H_2SO_4 solution and make up the volume to litre in volumetric flask.
2. Pipet out 0.1, 0.2, 0.3, 0.4, 0.5 to 1.0 ml from the above stock solution in 10 ml volumetric flasks and make up the volume with 0.5 M H_2SO_4 solution.

3. **Preparation of test sample:** Dissolve about 10 mg of the sample and dissolve in sufficient quantity of 0.5 M H_2SO_4 solution and make up the volume to litre in volumetric flask. Pipet out 0.4 ml from this solution in 10 ml volumetric flask and make up the volume with 0.5 M H_2SO_4 solution.

4. Follow the general direction provided by the teacher for the use of spectrofluorometer. Set the excitation wavelength to 350 nm and emission wavelength to 450 nm in the spectrofluorometer. Record the fluorescence intensity of all the ten standard solution by using sulfuric acid as blank solution.

5. Similarly, record the fluorescence intensity of sample solution.

Observation and calculation

Table. 11.1. Fluorescence intensity of quinine sulfate solution

S. No.	Concentration (µg)	Fluorescence intensity
1.	0.1	–
2.	0.2	–
3.	0.3	–
4.	0.4	–
5.	0.5	–
6.	0.6	–
7.	0.7	–
8.	0.8	–
9.	0.9	–
10.	1.0	–
11.	Unknown	–

Plot a calibration curve by plotting a graph between the concentration and emission intensity. Read out the concentration of unknown solution from the calibration curve. Multiply with dilution factor to get the concentration in the sample.

Result

The unknown solution contains .... mg/L.

Judge yourself

1. Define the terms 'fluorescence' and phosphorescence'.
2. Compare the absorption spectrum with the fluorescence spectrum. What are the similarities and differences?
3. What is quenching?
4. What is the excitation wavelength for quinine?

EXPERIMENT 48

Fluorimetric determination of riboflavin

Riboflavin is an important vitamin of the B complex (vitamin B_2) acting as an intermediary in the transfer of electrons in biological redox reactions and having an important function in cell growth. As with all vitamins of the B complex, riboflavin is the only one which is synthesized by microorganisms while others must be obtained from the food. Considering the high concentrations of B complex vitamins present in meat and milk, these foods are the best natural sources of riboflavin in the human diet.

Riboflavin

Experimental overview

Fluorescence excitation occurs by absorption of photons. It involves emission between states of the same multiplicity, usually singlet to singlet. As a consequence, fluorescence is short-lived, with luminescence ceasing almost immediately ($<10^{-5}$ s). One of the most attractive features of fluorescence method is their inherent sensitivity, with detection limits often being one to three orders of magnitude smaller than those encountered in absorption spectroscopy. Typical detection limits are in the parts per billion range.

An excitation spectrum is obtained by measuring luminescence intensity at a fixed wavelength while the excitation wavelength is varied. Because the first step in generation fluorescence emission is absorption of radiation to create excited states, an excitation spectrum is essentially identical to an absorbance spectrum taken under the same conditions. The excitation spectrum can be used to select appropriate wavelengths for excitation of fluorescence. Fluorescence and phosphorescence spectra (F and P, respectively), on the other hand, involve excitation at a fixed wavelength while recording the emission intensity as a function of wavelength. Usually radiation absorbed is converted with nearly constant quantum efficiency into fluorescence, and the absorption and excitation spectra are identical in every feature. Occasionally, the quantum efficiency for production of fluorescence varies with excitation wavelength, and small differences between the absorption and excitation spectra may be observed. The excitation spectrum should be used to obtain the optimum wavelength for excitation of fluorescence intensity.

In many applications, minimum sample treatment required because the native fluorescence properties of the analyte are used. For cases in which the analyte is not fluorescent or the fluorescence quantum efficiency is inadequate, derivatization reactions are used to convert the analyte into a product with good fluorescence characteristics. The fluorescence signal of the product is related to the analyte concentration. Most commonly, the analytical reaction is allowed to reach equilibrium before measurements are made.

In this experiment, prepare an accurate calibration curve of fluorescence intensity versus known concentration of riboflavin. These calibration curves will then be used to determine the concentration of a riboflavin solution that you will prepare.

Reagents required

1. Riboflavin (solid).
2. 10 µg/ml riboflavin standard.
3. 1% (v/v) acetic acid.
4. Unknown vitamin tablet.

Procedure

1. Using the stock riboflavin solution containing 10 µg/ml of riboflavin, prepare a series of ten standard solutions by dilutions with 1% (v/v) acetic acid solution. The strongest standard should not contain more than 1 µg/ml of riboflavin. The weakest standard solution should contain less than 0.1 µg/ml of riboflavin.
2. Set the excitation wavelength at 444 nm and emission wavelength at 520 nm. Take the fluorescent intensity of each standard dilution against the blank.
3. Weigh accurately 20 tablets and powder them. Prepare a solution by dissolving a weighed amount of powder equivalent to about 10 mg of riboflavin in 100 ml of 1% acetic acid solution.
4. Similarly, record the fluorescence intensity of the sample solution and determine the concentration of riboflavin in µg/ml.

Observation and calculation

Table 11.2. Fluorescence intensity of quinine sulfate solution

S. No.	Concentration (µg)	Fluorescence intensity
1.	0.1	–
2.	0.2	–
3.	0.3	–
4.	0.4	–
5.	0.5	–
6.	0.6	–
7.	0.7	–
8.	0.8	–
9.	0.9	–
10.	1.0	–
11.	Unknown	–

Plot a calibration curve by plotting a graph between the concentration and emission intensity. Read out the concentration of unknown solution from the calibration curve. Multiply with dilution factor to get the concentration in the sample.

Result

The average weight tablet contains .... mg of riboflavin.

Judge yourself

1. Explain why the radiation from fluorescence is measured 90° from the excitation radiation.
2. Discuss the other deactivation processes that compete with fluorescence.
3. Draw the structure of riboflavin. Discuss the structural features of the riboflavin molecule, which lead to its observed fluorescent properties.
4. Discuss the location and the intensity of peaks observed in your recorded spectra. What can you say about this spectral system?

EXPERIMENT 49

Fluorimetric determination of thiamine

Thiamine, also known as **vitamin B$_1$** and **aneurine hydrochloride**, is the term for a family of molecules sharing a common structural feature responsible for its activity as a vitamin. It is one of the B vitamins. Its most common form is a colorless chemical compound with a chemical formula $C_{12}H_{17}N_4OS$. Its chemical structure contains a pyrimidine ring and a thiazole ring. This form of thiamin is soluble in water, methanol, and glycerol and practically insoluble in acetone, ether, chloroform, and benzene.

Thiamine has essential metabolic roles in carbohydrate and protein metabolism and in neural function Common symptoms of thiamine deficiency often involve the nervous system and the heart. In less severe deficiency, nonspecific signs include malaise, weight loss, irritability and confusion.

Experimental overview

It is a non-fluorescent compound but can be assayed by fluorimetric method. It is quantitatively converted into fluorescent compound, thiochrome by alkaline potassium ferricyanide. The thiochrome (biologically inactive) is estimated by fluorimetric method.

Thiamine hydrochloride   Thiochrome

Reagents required

1. **Potassium ferricyanide (K$_3$Fe (CN)$_6$) solution:** Dissolve 1.0 g of potassium ferricyanide in 100 ml of water. Now mix 4 ml of the $K_3Fe(CN)_6$ solution with sufficient 15% w/v NaOH to make 100 ml of oxidizing reagent.
2. **Thiamine HCl stock solution:** Transfer 25 mg of thiamine HCl to a 1000 ml volumetric flask. Dissolve this in 300 ml of 20% C_2H_5OH which has been adjusted with 3 N HCl to a pH of 4.0. Now, add the acidified alcohol to make up the volume.

Procedure

1. To make the assay preparation, place in a suitable volumetric flask sufficient powder from the tablets to be assayed, such that when diluted to volume with 0.2 N HCl, the resulting solution will contain about 100 mg of thiamine HCl per ml. Now dilute 5 ml of this solution quantitatively and stepwise using 0.2 N HCl to an estimated concentration of 0.2 mg of thiamine HCl per ml.
2. Prepare the standard preparation by diluting a portion of the stock solution, quantitatively and stepwise, with 0.2 N HCl to obtain a preparation of 0.2 mg of thiamine HCl/ml.
3. The next step is to take three test tubes of about 40 ml capacity and pipet 5 ml of the standard preparation while quickly (within 2 seconds) adding 3 ml of the oxidizing reagent and 20 ml of isobutyl alcohol, mixing by vigorous shaking. Now prepare a blank of the standard

preparation in fourth test tube by substituting for the oxidizing agent an equal volume of the 15% NaOH and proceeding in the same manner.

Note: Thiochrome has more solubility in isobutyl alcohol.

4. Repeat this procedure on the standard preparation with the assay preparation by taking 3 test tubes, including the making of a blank.
5. Next, into each of eight test tubes, add 2 ml of 100% C_2H_5OH and allow the phases to separate.
6. Decant to draw off 10 ml of the clear supernatant isobutyl alcohol solution into standardized cells. Then measure the fluorescence in a suitable fluorometer having an input filter of narrow transmittance range with a maximum of 365 nm and an output filter with a maximum of about 465 nm.

Calculation

Calculate the mg of thiamine HCl in each 5 ml of the assay preparation using the formula:

$$\frac{A - b}{S - d}$$

in which A and S are the average fluorometer readings of the portion of the assay and standard preparation treated with the oxidizing reagent and b and d are the readings of the blanks of the assay preparation and standard preparation respectively.

Note: Calibration curve may also be obtained by taking different concentration of standard solution and then concentration of unknown solution is read from this curve.

Result

The amount of thiamine HCl is found to be .... mg.

Judge yourself

1. Why potassium ferricyanide is added in assay for thiamine?
2. What is role of thiamine in metabolic activities in body?
3. Why isobutyl alcohol is used?

Conductometric Titrations

Introduction

All the ions in a solution contribute to the electrical conductance of the solution. However, the contributions of different types of ions to electrical conductance differ, and the transport number of the ion measures the extent to which a given ion contributes to the electrical conductance of an electrolyte solution. Different ions have different transport numbers. Resolving the conductance of a solution to the contributions from the different types of ions is not very easy. Hence, conductance measurements is not a specific analytical method for the quantitative analysis of a given ion despite the fact conductance can be measured with high sensitivity (even the conductance of pure water, which is very low, can be measured precisely). Conductometry can, however, be used selectively to determine the amount of an electrolyte by following a titration in which the electrolyte participates. If the titration reaction involves a change of either the nature of the amount of ions then there will be a change of electrical conductance during the titration. In such cases, the titration may be followed conveniently, using conductometry. A titration carried out with the use of conductometry is known as a conductometric titration.

Consider a solution of a strong acid, hydrochloric acid, HCl for instance, to which a solution of a strong base, sodium hydroxide NaOH, is added. The reaction occurs. For each amount of NaOH added equivalent amount of hydrogen ions is removed. Effectively, the faster moving H^+ cation is replaced by the slower moving Na^+ ion, and the conductivity of the titrated solution as well as the measured conductance of the cell fall (Fig. 12.1). This continues until the equivalence point is reached, at which we have a solution of sodium chloride, NaCl. If more base is added an increase in conductivity or conductance is observed, since more ions are being added and the neutralization reaction no longer removes an appreciable number any of them. Consequently, in the titration of a strong acid with a strong base, the conductance has a minimum at the equivalence point. This minimum can be used instead of an indicator dye to determine the endpoint of the titration.

Conductometric titration curve is a plot of the measured conductance or conductivity values against the number of milliliters of NaOH solution.

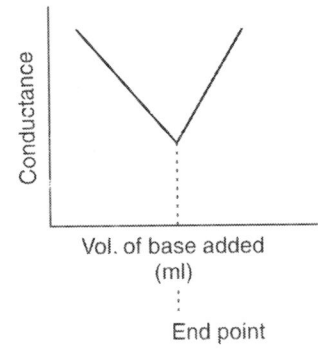

Vol. of base added
(ml)

End point

Fig. 12.1

EXPERIMENT 50

Conductometric titration of hydrochloric acid and acetic acid with sodium hydroxide

Experimental overview

Conductance (G) is the reciprocal of electrical resistance (R).

$$G = \frac{1}{R}$$

It is a measure of the ability of a solution to conduct electricity. The conductance of a solution is the sum of the conductances of all of the ions that are in the solution.

$$G = \Sigma G \text{ ions}$$

The conductance of a particular ion in solution depends upon the concentration of the ion, the charge on the ion, and the size of the ion. As the concentration or the charge of the ion increases, the conductance of the solution increases. In general as the size of the solvated ion decreases, its mobility through the solution increases and consequently the conductance of the solution increases. In water, the ion which has the greatest conductance is H^+. Of the common, negative ions, OH^- has the greatest conductance. The relative conductances (relative to acetate) of the species that are involved in the experiment are listed in the Table 12.1.

Molecular species (uncharged substances) do not contribute to the conductance of a solution.

Table 12.1. Relative conductances of the various species

Species	Relative conductance
H^+	8.5
OH^-	4.8
Cl^-	1.9
Na^+	1.2
$C_2H_3O_2^-$	1.0
$HC_2H_3O_2$	0
H_2O	0

During the titration of hydrochloric acid with sodium hydroxide, the reaction that takes place in the titration vessel is

$$H^- + Cl^- \xrightarrow{\quad Na^+ \ OH^- \quad} H_2O + Cl^- + Na^+$$

Before the endpoint, H^+ is removed from the solution by reaction with OH^-, and Na^+ is added to the solution. Since the relative conductance of H+ is about seven times that of Na^+, the conductance of the solution decreases prior to the endpoint.

After the endpoint, no H^+ is available to react, and the conductance of the solution increases as a result of the addition of Na^+ and OH^-. Consequently the titration curve has a V-shape as shown below in the figure. The endpoint of the titration corresponds to the intersection of the extrapolated linear portions of the titration curve.

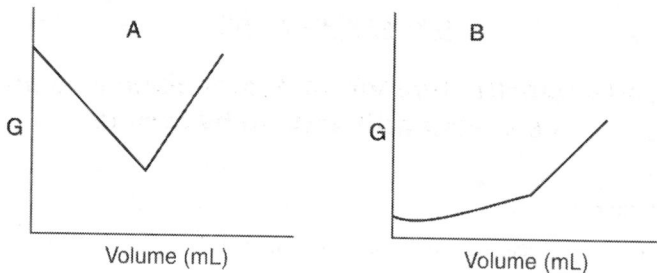

Volume (mL)   Volume (mL)

Fig. 12.2: Conductometric titration curves. A, the titration of HCl with NaOH; B, the titration of $HC_2H_3O_2$ with NaOH.

Since acetic acid is dissociated slightly (Ka = 1.8×10^{-5}) in aqueous solution, the conductance of the acetic acid solution is initially small. As sodium hydroxide is added, the hydroxide reacts with the acid to form water and acetate.

$$HC_2H_3O_2 \xrightarrow{\quad Na^+,\, OH^- \quad} H_2O + Na^+ + C_2H_3O_2^-$$
$$\Updownarrow$$
$$H^+ + C_2H_3O_2^-$$

The addition of $C_2H_3O_2^-$ and Na^+ to the solution causes the conductance of the solution to increase. After the endpoint, Na^+ and OH^- are added to the solution. Since the relative conductance of OH^- is nearly five times that of $C_2H_3O_2^-$, the conductance of the solution after the endpoint increases more rapidly than it did before the endpoint. The endpoint corresponds to the intersection of the extrapolated linear portions of the curve.

Conductance is usually measured with an alternating current between two identical, platinized platinum electrodes. Use of an alternating current prevents the buildup of reaction products around either electrode and consequently prevents polarization of the solution. The electrodes must be rigidly held at a fixed distance apart during the titrations in order to prevent changes in conductance that result from an altered solution volume between the electrodes.

Reagents required

1. Potassium hydrogen phthalate.
2. NaOH.
3. Acetic acid.
4. HCl solution.

Procedure

1. Dry the potassium hydrogen phthalate in a 110°C oven for at least 1 hour. After the drying period remove the compound from the oven and allow it to cool to room temperature in a desiccator.
2. Prepare 0.1 M NaOH solution by dissolving 4 g of NaOH in 1 litre of water.
3. Weigh to the nearest 0.1 mg, between 0.7 and 0.9 g of the dried potassium hydrogen phthalate into each of three, labeled, 250 ml Erlenmeyer flasks. Record the mass of the solid that is in each flask.

4. Add 30 ml of distilled or deionized water and two drops of phenolphthalein solution to each flask. Fill the 50 ml buret with the sodium hydroxide solution. Titrate the solution which is in each Erlenmeyer flask to the endpoint with the sodium hydroxide solution. The endpoint color change is from colorless to light pink. Record the three endpoint volumes to the nearest 0.01 ml.

5. Obtain at least 35 ml of an acetic acid solution and at least 35 ml of a hydrochloric acid solution from the instructor. Record the sample numbers.

6. Use a pipet to add 10 ml of the hydrochloric acid solution to the 250 ml, tall-form beaker. Add about 140 ml of distilled or deionized water and a stirring bar to the beaker. Place the beaker on a magnetic stirrer. Use a clamp to suspend the electrodes in the solution. The platinum electrodes must be completely submerged in the solution, but they should not interfere with operation of the stirring bar. Adjust the stirring rate to yield a smoothly stirred solution.

7. Refill the buret with sodium hydroxide solution. Measure the initial conductance of the stirred solution. Add 1 ml portions of the sodium hydroxide solution to the stirred solution. Record the conductance of the titrant solution and the total volume (to the nearest 0.01 ml) of the added titrant solution after each addition. Continue the titration until the endpoint has been passed by 100%, i.e. until a total volume that is twice the endpoint volume has been added.

8. Similarly dilute and titrate two, more 10 ml portions of the hydrochloric acid solution, and three, 10 ml portions of the acetic acid solution.

9. After the titrations have been completed, store the electrodes in water.

Observation and calculations

a) **For acetic acid solution:**

S. No.	Vol of NaOH	Conductance
1.	–	–
2.	–	–
3.	–	–
4.	–	–
5.	–	–
6.	–	–

b) **For HCl solution:**

S. No.	Vol of NaOH	Conductance
1.	–	–
2.	–	–
3.	–	–
4.	–	–
5.	–	–
6.	–	–

1. Use the mass of potassium hydrogen phthalate (MW 204.23) that was in each flask and the corresponding endpoint volume of the sodium hydroxide solution to calculate three values of the concentration (M) of the sodium hydroxide solution.

2. For each conductometric titration, plot conductance (y axis) as a function of the volume of the added sodium hydroxide solution. Draw a straight line through each of the two, linear portions in each titration curve. Determine the endpoint volume of each titration from the intersection of the two straight lines.

3. Use the endpoint volumes and the mean sodium hydroxide concentration to calculate three values of the concentration of the original hydrochloric acid solution and three values of the concentration of the original acetic acid solution.

Result

The strength of acetic acid and hydrochloric acid is found to be .... and .... respectively.

Judge yourself

1. What is specific conductance?
2. Mention the factor affecting the conductance.
3. Why the concentration decreases initially in conductometric titration of acetic acid with NaOH solution?
4. Mention the various methods of detecting the endpoints in titrations.
5. What is over-titration?

13

Thin Layer Chromatography

Introduction

Chromatography is a sophisticated method of separating mixtures of two or more compounds. The separation is accomplished by the distribution of the mixture between two phases—one that is stationary and one that is moving. Chromatography works on the principle that different compounds will have different solubilities and adsorption to the two phases between which they are to be partitioned.

Thin Layer Chromatography (TLC) is a solid-liquid technique in which the two phases are a solid (stationary phase) and a liquid (moving phase). Solids most commonly used in chromatography are silica gel ($SiO_2 \times H_2O$) and alumina ($Al_2O_3 \times H_2O$). Both of these adsorbents are polar, but alumina is more so. Silica is also acidic. Alumina is available in neutral, basic, or acidic forms. TLC is a sensitive, fast, simple and inexpensive analytical technique. It is a micro technique; as little as 10^{-9} g of material can be detected, although the sample size is from 1 to 100×10^{-6} g. TLC involves spotting the sample to be analyzed near one end of a sheet of glass or plastic that is coated with a thin layer of an adsorbent. The sheet, which can be the size of a microscope slide, is placed in a covered jar containing a shallow layer of solvent. As the solvent rises by capillary action up through the adsorbent, differential partitioning occurs between the components of the mixture dissolved in the solvent the stationary adsorbent phase. The more strongly a given component of a mixture is adsorbed onto the stationary phase, the less time it will spend in the mobile phase and the more slowly it will migrate up the plate.

Visualization of compounds

There are various techniques to visualize the compounds on TLC plate.

1. Sulfuric acid/heat: destructive, leaves charred blots behind
2. Ceric stain: destructive, leaves a dark blue blot behind for polar compounds
3. Iodine: semi-destructive, iodine absorbs onto the spots, not permanent
4. UV light: non-destructive, long wavelength (background green, spots dark), short wavelength (plate dark, compounds glow).

The following are some common uses of thin layer chromatography.

1. To determine the number of components in a mixture.
2. To determine the identity of two substances.
3. To monitor the progress of a reaction.
4. To determine the effectiveness of a purification.
5. To determine the appropriate conditions for a column chromatographic separation.
6. To monitor column chromatography.

EXPERIMENT 51

Identification of given unknown drug by using thin layer chromatography

Experimental overview

Thin Layer Chromatography (TLC) is one of the methods available for the separation and tentative identification of components present in mixtures. A compound will travel at a fixed rate depending on its relative solubility in a moving solvent and retaining capacity of the stationary phase. The stationary phase in TLC is the silica gel or other solid material. The moving phase is a solvent system that will dissolve some of the components of the mixture more readily than others.

A solution of the mixture to be analyzed is spotted on a thin layer plate and then the lower edge of the plate is placed into the solvent system. The solvent moves up the plate carrying with it any components that are dissolved in it. The distance the components are carried up the plate depends on how soluble each component is in the solvent and how much interaction or attraction the component has for the stationary phase. The more soluble the component is in the solvent, the farther the component travels. The more interactions the component has with the silica gel on the thin layer plate, the less distance it will travel.

The location of each component must be determined by making them visible, if they are not already visible. This may require a visualizer, which can be a chemical or an instrument.

The distance that the component has traveled is normally recorded by computing an 'R_f' value (Relative flow value) (Fig. 13.1). This value is calculated by applying the following formula.

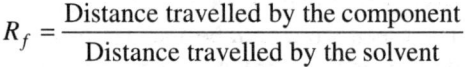

$$R_f = \frac{\text{Distance travelled by the component}}{\text{Distance travelled by the solvent}}$$

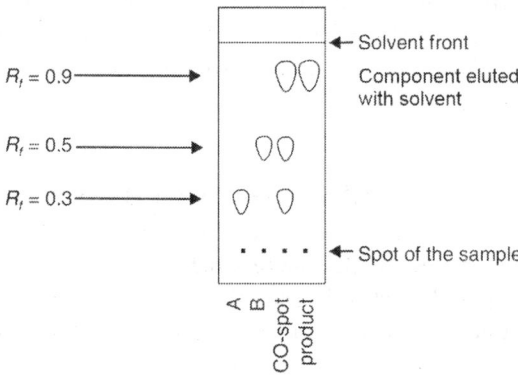

Fig. 13.1: Example of thin layer chromatography.

This R_f is characteristic of the substance in the solvent system used and helps identify the unknown substance. The size of the spot provides a rough quantitative measure of the amount of the substance present.

When you work with a particular group of compounds, 'known samples' should be run with the unknown to avoid any uncertainties caused by variations in the system, as well as for comparison purposes at the time of identification.

Procedure

1. Obtain a thin layer chromatographic plate containing stationary phase (silica gel G). Contamination and damage to the surface of the plate may be avoided by holding the plate at the edges.

2. Using a pencil only, draw a baseline, approximately 1.5 cm from the bottom of the plate. Mark seven equidistant spots on this baseline, and label them 1, 2, 3, 4, 5, unknown, and Mixture. Put your initials on the plate, in pencil, in order to be able to distinguish your plate from those of your classmates.

3. Obtain six clean dry test tubes and label them using a marker, as follows:
   Test tube 1: Caffeine (a stimulant).
   Test tube 2: Ibuprofen (an analgesic).
   Test tube 3: Phenacetin (an analgesic).
   Test tube 4: Quinine (an antimalarial).
   Test tube 5: Salicylic acid (an analgesic).
   Test tube 6: Unknown sample.

4. To each of the tubes labeled above add a spatula-tip full of the appropriate drug, in its powdered form. Be sure to avoid contamination from one tube to the next.
   Tube 6: This is an unknown sample that you have to identify using the technique of thin layer chromatography. The instructor will provide you with this sample. It should be treated exactly the same as the standard (known) drugs.

5. In the hood, add approximately 3 ml of concentrated ammonium hydroxide to each tube, and mix gently (**Caution:** Do not inhale the ammonium hydroxide fumes). Then, add 1 ml of the ethyl acetate solvent to each tube and mix thoroughly. Let the tubes stand for a few minutes in order to allow the ammonium hydroxide and the ethyl acetate to separate (use a centrifuge if necessary).

6. Using a clean dropper for each tube, transfer a portion of the upper (ethyl acetate) layer to a clean, labeled tube. Be careful not to transfer any of the ammonium hydroxide layer.

7. Using a new capillary tube for each sample, spot each of the samples on the appropriate mark on the chromatography plate. Some samples may have to be spotted more than once. Let the spots dry. To the mark labeled 'mixture' on the plate, spot one drop of each of the five standard drugs. To the mark labeled 'unknown' on the plate, spot the unknown sample from Tube 6 a few times.

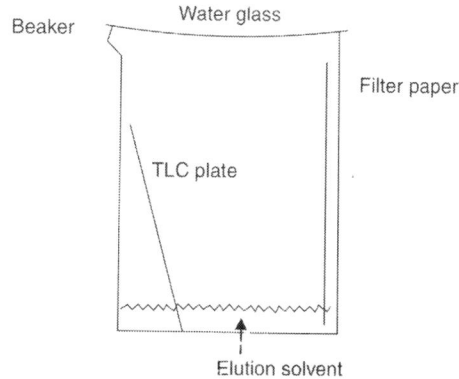

Fig. 13.2

8. Prepare a solvent chamber with solvent system. The solvent system is a mixture of ethyl acetate : methanol : ammonium hydroxide (85 : 10 : 5). Place a sufficient solvent system in the chamber. Place a filter paper along the wall of the chamber. Keep it for 5 to 10 minutes to provide the inner atmosphere saturated with solvent vapors.

9. Place the plate in the prepared 'solvent chamber' located in the hood. The spot of drug, applied on TLC plate should not be dipped into the solvent system. When the solvent has moved 3/4 of the way up the plate, remove the plate. Let it dry in the hood.

10. Examine your plate under short wavelength ultraviolet light in order to visualize your results. Be sure to check the origin for any drugs that do not readily move in the solvent. Spots of the compounds can also be visualized by keeping the TLC plate in iodine chamber.

Observation

Diagram your observations on the Report Sheet. Calculate the R_f value of each drug and identify the unknown drug.

Result

The unknown drug is found to be ... .

Judge yourself

1. What is relative flow rate?
2. What is the principle of thin layer chromatography?
3. Why silica gel G is used as stationary phase?
4. How mobile phase is selected?

14

Paper Chromatography

Introduction

Paper chromatography is an analytical technique for separating and identifying mixtures that are or can be colored, especially pigments. This can also be used in secondary or primary colors in ink experiments. This method has been largely replaced by thin layer chromatography, however it is still a powerful teaching tool. **Two-way paper chromatography**, also called **two-dimensional chromatography**, involves using two solvents and rotating the paper 90° in between. This is useful for separating complex mixtures of similar compounds, for example, amino acids.

A small concentrated spot of solution that contains the sample of the solute is applied to a strip of chromatography paper about two centimeters away from the base of the plate, usually using a capillary tube for maximum precision. This sample is absorbed onto the paper and may form interact with it. Any substance that reacts or bonds with the paper cannot be measured using this technique. The paper is then dipped into a suitable solvent, such as ethanol or water, taking care that the spot is above the surface of the solvent, and placed in a sealed container. The solvent moves up the paper by capillary action, which occurs as a result of the attraction of the solvent molecules to the paper, also this can be explained as differential adsorption of the solute components into the solvent. As the solvent rises through the paper it meets and dissolves the sample mixture, which will then travel up the paper with the solvent solute sample. Different compounds in the sample mixture travel at different rates due to differences in solubility in the solvent, and due to differences in their attraction to the fibers in the paper. Paper chromatography takes anywhere from several minutes to several hours. In some cases, paper chromatography does not separate pigments completely; this occurs when two substances appear to have the same values in a particular solvent. In these cases, two-way chromatography is used to separate the multiple-pigment spots.

Ascending chromatography

In this method, the solvent is in pool at the bottom of the vessel in which the paper is supported. It rises up the paper by capillary action against the force of gravity.

Descending chromatography

In this method, the solvent is kept in a trough at the top of the chamber and is allowed to flow down the paper. The liquid moves down by capillary action as well as by the gravitational force. In this case, the flow is more rapid as compared to the ascending method. Because of this rapid speed, the chromatography is completed in a comparatively shorter time. The apparatus needed for this case is more sophisticated. The developing solvent is placed in a trough at the top which is usually made up of an inert material. The paper is then suspended in the solvent. Substances that cannot be separated by ascending method, can be separated by the above descending method.

Detection

After development, the spots corresponding to different compounds may be located by their color, ultraviolet light, ninhydrin (triketohydrindane hydrate) or by treatment with iodine vapors. The paper remaining after the experiment is known as the chromatogram. The components which have been separated differ in their retention factor i.e Ratio of distance traveled from the spot or origin by the solute component to that of the distance traveled from the spot or origin by the solvent. Retention Factor can never be greater than one. To calculate Rf, use the following.

$$R_f = \frac{\text{Distance travelled by sample}}{\text{Distance travelled by solvent}}$$

The final chromatogram can be compared with other known **mixture** chromatograms to identify sample mixes using the Rf value in an experiment. The retention values found can be compared to known values, and from that conclusions can be drawn.

R_f value

R_f value may be defined as the ratio of the distance travelled by the substance to the distance travelled by the solvent. R_f values are usually expressed as a fraction of two decimal places. If R_f value of a solution is zero, the solute remains in the stationary phase and thus it is immobile. If R_f value = 1, then the solute has no affinity for the stationary phase and travels with the solvent front.

EXPERIMENT 52

Chromatographic separation and identification of sugars

Experimental overview

The term chromatography comes from the earlier times when the technique was used for the separation of colored plants pigments. Chromatography is a technique for separation of closely related groups of compounds. The separation is brought about by differential migration along a porous medium and the migration is caused by the flow of solvent.

Within limits chromatography can be divided into two types: partition and adsorption chromatography. Paper chromatography is an example of partition chromatography.

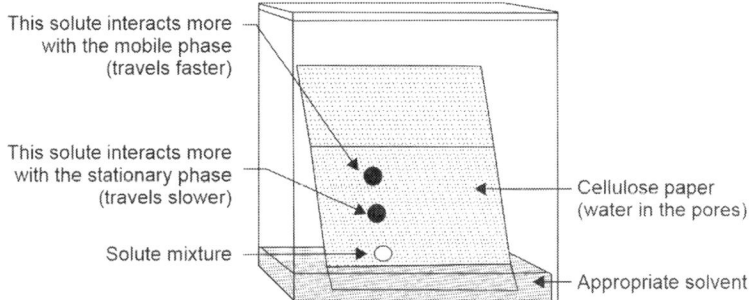

Fig. 14.1: Illustrative scheme for paper chromatography.

In this type of chromatography, separation is due to differential partition of solutes between two liquid phases (Fig. 14.1). One liquid phase is bound to the porous medium for example, the water bound in the cellulose paper, this phase is referred to as, the stationary phase. The other liquid phase, the mobile phase flows along the porous medium. As the mobile phase flows over the solute mixture, the individual solutes partition themselves between the aqueous stationary phase and the organic mobile phase relative to their solubilities in the two phases. The more soluble a solute in the mobile phase, the faster it will travel along the paper, and conversely, the mobile phase must be a mixture in which the compounds to be separated are soluble or partially soluble. In paper chromatography solute or solute mixture is spotted in solution along a base line on a sheet of filter paper (Whatman No. 1). The mobile phase (solvent) is allowed to flow over the spots either ascending the paper by capillary action or descending the paper by gravity.

The separation is measured in terms of a unit called R_f (relative rates of flow) with respect to the solvent front. Fig. 14.2 explains how to calculate this value.

The R_f value of a compound in a particular solvent system is constant under identical conditions of the experiment, e.g. temperature, pH, etc.

Because most compound are colorless the spots are visualized after separation by specific reagent. The location reagent is applied by spraying the paper or rapidly dipping it in a solution of the reagent in a volatile solvent. Viewing under ultraviolet light is also useful since some compound which absorb it strongly show up as dark spots against the florescent background of the paper.

Reagents required

Paper: Usually Whatman No. 1 filter paper is used because of its known grade.

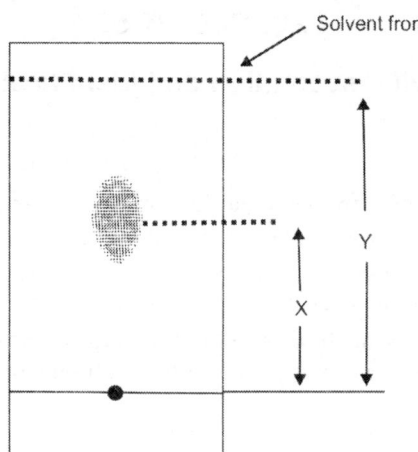

Fig. 14.2: $R_f = \dfrac{X}{Y} = \dfrac{\text{Distance moved by the sample}}{\text{Distance moved by the solvent}}$

Solvents (either of these):

(a) Water-saturated phenol + 1% ammonia.

(b) *n*-butanol-acetic acid-water (4:1:5 v/v).

(c) Isopropanol–pyridine–water–acetic acid (8:8:4:1 v/v).

Note: Use of *n*-butanol system is more common.

Spray reagents

a. **Ammoniacal silver nitrate:** Add equal volumes of NH_4OH to a saturated solution of $AgNO_3$ and dilute the methanol to give a final concentration of 0.3 M. After spraying the developed chromatograms, place them in an oven for 5–10 minutes, when the reducing sugars appear as brown spots.

b. **Alkaline permanganate:** Prepare aqueous solution of $KMNO_4$ (1%) containing 2% Na_2CO_3. After spraying with this mixture, the chromatograms are kept at 100°C for a few minutes, when the sugar spots appear as yellow spots in purple background.

c. **Aniline hydrogen phthalate:** Dissolve 1 ml of aniline and 1.66 g of phthalic acid in 100 ml of 1-butanol saturated with water.

d. **Resorcinol reagent:** Mix 1% ethanolic solution of resorcinol and 0.2 N HCl (1:1 v/v). Spray the dried chromatograms and visualize spots by heating at 90°C.

Procedure

1. Place sufficient solvent into the bottom of the tank. Cover the led and allow the tank to be saturated with the solvent.

2. Take a sheet of Whatman No. 1 chromatography paper (about 9 × 10 cm) and place it on a piece of clean paper on a bench.

3. Draw a fine line with a pencil along the width of the paper and about 1.5 cm from the lower edge.

4. Along this line place four equality spaced (about 2 cm apart) small circles with a pencil.

5. Label the paper at the top with the name of each of the sugars and label the last unknown.

6. Use a fine capillary or tooth pick to place the drops of the solutions of the sugars, glucose, fructose, maltose, lactose and the mixture.

7. After spotting, dry the paper with hot air dryer for one minute, repeat this step again.

8. Place the spotted paper in the chromatographic tank and make the development by using the ascending technique.

9. Close the tank with lid, allow the solvent to flow for about 30–45 minutes.

10. Remove the paper and immediately mark the position of the solvent front with a pencil.

11. After the chromatogram has dried, spray the paper with the locating reagent.

12. Dry at low temperature or expose it to the hot air dryer, until the colored spots appear. The colors are stable for some weeks if kept in the dark and away from acid vapors.

13. Circle the position of each colored spot with pencil.

Observation and calculation

General summary of the behavior of the various sugars to these reagents is given below:

Sugars	a	b	c	d
Aldohexoses	+	+	+	Pink
Ketohexoses	+	+	+	Red
Aldopentoses	+	+	+	Blue, green
Ketopentoses	+	+	+	–
Deoxy sugars	–	+	+	–
Glycosides	+	–	–	–
Amino sugars	+	+	+	–

Calculate the R_f value for each spot and also for the spots the mixture contained.

The table below R_f values of some sugars in the solvents previously mentioned. They are only for comparative purposes, since R_f varies with physical parameters.

Sugar	Solvent a	Solvent b	Solvent c
Glucose	0.39	0.18	0.64
Galactose	0.44	0.16	0.62
Fructose	0.51	0.25	0.68
Ribose	0.59	0.31	0.76
Deoxy ribose	0.73	–	–
Lactose	0.38	0.09	0.46
Maltose	0.36	0.11	0.50
Sucrose	0.39	0.14	0.62

Result

1. Draw a sketch of your chromatogram.

2. By comparing the R_f values of the mixture along with those for the standards, state what sugars does this mixture contain.

The popular detecting agent is aniline hydrogen phthalate. In this, heating of sugar with an acid produces furfuraldehyde which can be condensed with an aromatic amine to give colored compounds. Sugar which reacts can appear as red or brown spots.

Judge yourself

1. What is partition chromatography? Mention with example.
2. What is R_f value? How it is calculated?
3. Why sulfuric acid is not used as spray reagent in paper chromatography?
4. Classify the various techniques of paper chromatography.

UV-Visible Absorbance Spectroscopy

Introduction

In molecular absorbance spectroscopy, a beam of ultraviolet or visible light is directed through a sample. Some of the light may be transmitted through the sample (Fig. 15.1). Light that was not transmitted through the sample was absorbed. Transmittance (T) is defined as the ratio of P and P_0.

Absorbance (A) is defined as $-\log (T)$.

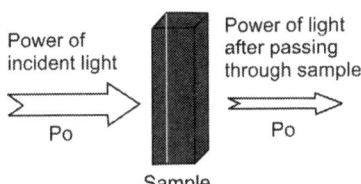

Power of incident light

Power of light after passing through sample

Po

Po

Sample

Fig. 15.1

A molecule can absorb some of the light only if it can accommodate that additional energy by promoting electrons to higher energy levels (Fig. 15.2). The energy of the light being absorbed must match the energy required to promote the electron. Therefore, not all wavelengths of light are absorbed equally by a sample. An absorbance spectrum depicts what wavelengths of light are absorbed by a sample. The UV-visible absorbance spectrum below was obtained by passing different wavelengths of light through a solution of fabric dye, and measuring the intensity of light (P) passing through the solution. One can readily see what wavelengths of light are absorbed (peaks), and what wavelenghts of light are transmitted (troughs).

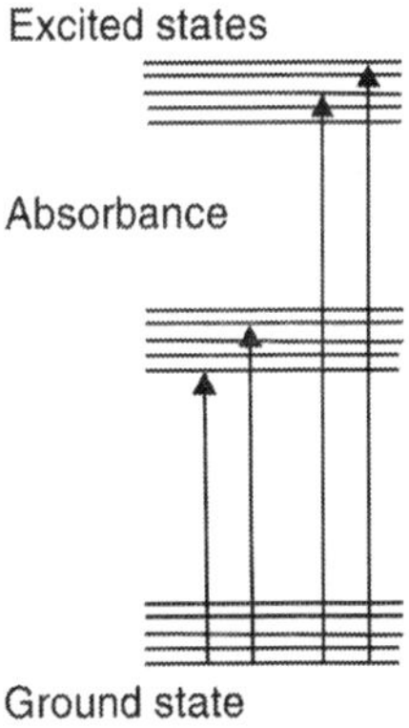

One very important relationship in absorbance spectroscopy is **Beer's law:**

$$A = abc$$

where A = absorbance

a = molar absorptivity, describes the ability of a molecule to absorb radiation at a particular wavelength

b = length of sample through which the light beam passes

c = concentration of the absorbing species

Excited states

Absorbance

Ground state

Fig. 15.2

This relationship (Fig. 15.3) is the basis of all quantitative work in absorbance spectroscopy. It allows one to determine the concentration of an absorbing species simply by measuring its absorbance.

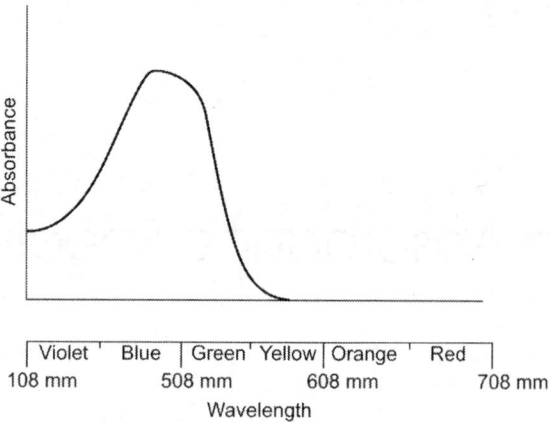

Fig. 15.3: Absorbance spectrum of a dye.

EXPERIMENT 53

Determination of λ_{max} of chlorpheniramine maleate, absorptivity, molar absorptivity and specific absorbance

Chlorpheniramine maleate occurs as an odorless, white, crystalline powder with a melting point between 130–135°C and a pKa of 9.2. One gram is soluble in about 4 ml of water, or 10 ml of alcohol. The pH of the commercially available injection is between 4–5.2.

Chlorpheniramine maleate is an antihistamine that blocks the effects of the naturally occurring histamine in body. It is used to treat sneezing; runny nose; itching, watery eyes; hives; rashes; itching; and other symptoms of allergies and the common cold.

Chlorpheniramine maleate

Experimental overview

When a light beam passes through a glass cuvette containing liquid, the emergent radiation is less powerful than that entering mainly because of "absorption" of radiant energy by the liquid. However, reflections at the cuvette surfaces and scattering by suspended particles (if any) also decrease emergent radiation intensity. The absorption occurs not only in visible region but also in UV and infrared ranges.

Beer's (or sometimes known as Beer-Lambert's) law explains the absorption of radiant energy by matter. When the losses by reflection at the cuvette surfaces and absorption by the cuvette (glass) are neglected; the radiation diminishes in power proportionally with the number of absorbing molecules in the path of the beam. The Beer's law states:

"Successive increments in the number of identical absorbing molecules in the path of a beam of monochromatic radiation absorb equal fractions of the radiant energy traversing them".

$A = \log (P_o/P) = a\,b\,c$

$P =$ radiant power; $P_o =$ initial radiant power

$A =$ absorbance; (property of a particular sample; an extensive property)

$a =$ absorptivity; (a characteristic of a particular combination of solute and solvent for a given wavelength; property of a substance. If the nature of the absorbing material hence its molecular weight is known, a can be converted to molar absorptivity (extinction coefficient), ε);

$b =$ length of path; (customarily in centimeters)

$c =$ concentration (g/L)

Reagents required

1. Chlorpheniramine maleate.
2. 0.1 M hydrochloric acid.

Procedure

1. **Preparation of stock solution of chlorpheniramine maleate:** Dissolve 0.1 g of chlorpheniramine maleate in 50 ml of 0.1 MHCl solution.
3. **Preparation of standard solution of chlorpheniramine maleate:** Dilute 10 ml of stock solution to 100 ml with 0.1 M HCl solution (0.005 g/100 ml or 0.05 g/Litre).
3. Measure the absorbance of the chlorpheniramine maleate solution.

Observation and calculation

Absorbance of chlorpheniramine maleate solution at different wavelength

Wavelength (nm)	Absorbance
240	0.529
250	0.582
255	0.677
260	0.831
265	**1.005**
270	0.913
280	0.496
290	0.128

According to Beer-Lambert law:

$$A = abc$$

A = Absorbance, a = molar absorptivity, b = path length, c = concentration

$$1.005 = a \times 1 \times 0.05$$

(i) Absorptivity (a) = 1.005/0.05 = 20.1
(ii) Molar absorptivity
   Conc./mol. wt. = mole/litre
   0.05/340 = 0.00015 mole/litre
   $A = a \times b \times c$
   $1.005 = a \times 1 \times 0.00015$
   $a = 6700$
(iii) Specific absorbance
   A (1%, 1 cm) = a/c = 1.005/0.005 = 201

Result

(i) λ_{max} = 265 nm.
(ii) Absorptivity = 20.1.
(iii) Molar absorptivity = 6700.
(iv) Specific absorbance = 201.

Judge yourself

1. Which wavelength of visible light possesses the greatest energy value, and what is its color?
2. Which wavelength possesses the least energy value, and what is its color?
3. What is transmittance?
4. In which unit wavelength is measured?

EXPERIMENT 54

Spectrophotometric determination of acetylsalicylic acid content in aspirin tablet

Experimental view

Acetylsalicylic acid, the active ingredient in aspirin, can be analyzed by quantitatively converting it to salicylate ion, which is complexed with Fe^{+3}. The iron-salicylate complex absorbs green light, and can be quantitated using absorption spectrometry.

Acetylsalicylic acid can be hydrolyzed with NaOH to form the salicylate dianion as follows:

The salicylate dianion complexes with many transition metal cations including Fe^{+3}:

In this experiment, the acetylsalicylic acid in commercial tablets will be converted to the iron-salicylate complex and that will be quantitated by measuring its absorbance.

The absorbance of a series of standard iron-salicylate solutions will be measured to calibrate the absorption spectrometer. The concentration of the unknown iron-salicylate solution will be used to find the percent acetylsalicylic acid in the original tablets.

Comments: The pH of the solution in which the complexation reaction is run must be kept between 0.5 and 2.0. If the pH gets too high the iron will precipitate out as a hydroxide and if the pH is too low the salicylate dianions will be protonated rendering them unavailable to the complexation reaction. The pH is controlled with hydrochloric acid.

Reagents required

1. Concentrated HCl solution
2. 1 M NaOH
3. 0.025 M $FeCl_3$ solution. Add 6.8 g $FeCl_3.6H_2O$ to100 ml deionized water in a 250 ml beaker. Add 3.0 ml of concentrated HCl and 12.0 g of KCl. Dissolve and dilute to 1.0 L with deionized water.

Procedure

1. **Stock salicylate solution:** Weigh accurately about 0.4 g of acetylsalicylic acid and place it into 100 ml Erlenmeyer flask. Add 10 ml of 1.0 M NaOH and heat the mixture to boiling. Boil for five minutes and avoid splattering, washing down the sides of the flask with deionized

water as needed. Cool and quantitatively transfer this solution to a 500 ml volumetric flask, and dilute to the mark with water.

2. **Standard iron-salicylate solutions**: Place the stock salicylate solution in a 50 ml buret. Deliver 10.00 ml of stock solution to your 100 ml volumetric flask. Dilute to the mark with 0.025 M $FeCl_3$ solution. Transfer the solution to a sealable bottle, rinsing the bottle with three 5 ml portions of the solution before transferring. Rinse the flask at least three times with deionized water before making the next standard solution.

   Repeat the above procedure four more times by transferring 8.00, 6.00, 4.00, and 2.00 ml to the volumetric flask. Be sure to record each volume to 0.01 ml and to label each bottle.

3. **Preparation of aspirin unknown solutions:** Weigh accurately 20 aspirin tablet and find out the average weight. Powder them. Transfer the powder equivalent to 0.3 g of aspirin into 100 ml erlenmeyer flasks and hydrolyze them the same way you hydrolyzed the acetylsalicylic acid as done in making standards solution. Dilute each one to 500.0 ml with deionized water. Transfer 10.00 ml of this solution to the 100 ml volumetric flask and dilute to the mark with $FeCl_3$ solution. Transfer each solution to a labeled bottle.

4. Read the absorbance of the highest concentration standard by measuring the absorbance at a wavelength of 530 nm. Use $FeCl_3$ solution as the blank solution.

   Make a plot of absorbance vs. wavelength and draw a smooth curve through the data points. Similarly, measure the absorbance of the unknown solutions again using $FeCl_3$ as the blank solution.

Observation and calculation

1. Make a calibration curve [absorbance vs concentration] from the standard solution data. Use the standard iron–salicylate concentrations for the calibration curve.

Table 15.1: Absorbance value at λ 530 nm

S. No.	Solution	Absorbance
1. Std	2 ml	–
2. Std	4 ml	–
3. Std	6 ml	–
4. Std	8 ml	–
5. Std	10 ml	–
6. Unknown	–	
7. Unknown	–	
8. Unknown	–	

2. Average the three unknown absorbance values and use that average with the analytical function [from the calibration curve] to calculate the average concentration of iron-salicylate in the unknown solutions. Also calculate the standard deviation in the concentration.

3. Use the average iron-salicylate concentration and the average tablet mass to calculate the average w/w % acetylsalicylic acid in the original tablet.

Result

The amount of acetylsalicylic acid/average weight tablet is ..... mg.

Judge yourself

1. At what pH salicylate form complex with ferric chloride?
2. What is the systematic name of aspirin?
3. What is the best solvent for aspirin?
4. There are various methods for quantitative determination of acetylsalicylic acid content. Which method is the most accurate?
5. Why acetylsalicylic acid does not form complex with ferric chloride?

EXPERIMENT 55

Determination of salicylic acid (%) in synthesized aspirin by spectrophotometric method

Experimental view

The purity of the synthesized aspirin can be tested by addition of Fe^{+3} to a suspension of the product. Phenols (such as salicylic acid) react with ferric chloride to form colored complex. The complex formed between Fe^{3+} ion and salicylic acid is blue, which allows its visual detection. Obviously, the intensity of the observed color is proportional to the complex concentration. Complex concentration can be determined by Spectrophotometric measurement of the absorbance of the complex in the visible region (at 540 nm). The Beer-Lambert law states that the proportion of light absorbed by a solute in a transparent solvent is proportional to the number of absorbing molecules in the light path.

$$A = \varepsilon bc$$

where:

A = absorbance
ε = molar absorptivity
b = cell (path) length (cm)
c = sample concentration (in mol/L)

Therefore, the absorbance is in direct relation with the concentration of the absorbent species.

The concentration can be determined by measuring the absorbance of the sample. Several solutions of salicylic acid of known concentration must be prepared, and their absorbance measured at the desired wavelength. A plot of absorbance versus concentration gives standard curve.

The $FeCl_3$ solution is added to a sample of aspirin impurified with salicylic acid to form complex. Absorbance of the solution is determined. The concentration of the complex, and therefore the purity of the aspirin, will be calculated from the standard curve.

Reagents required

1. 5% $FeCl_3$ (aq) solution.
2. 0.2 M salicylic acid solution (mol. wt. = 138) (in ethanol).

Procedure

Qualitative determination of the residual salicylic acid

The purity of the synthesized aspirin can be tested by addition of Fe^{+3} to a suspension of the product. Prepare a tube with a small amount (a few crystals) of aspirin. Add water (2 ml) and 1 ml of 0.1 % aqueous solution of $FeCl_3$. The color development is considered a positive test and is an indication of the presence of free salicylic acid.

Quantitative determination of the residual salicylic acid by spectrophotometry

1. **Preparation of the calibration curve:** A series of standard complex solutions will be prepared, and their absorbance measured at 540 nm in a spectrophotometer. Concentrations of solutions must be ranged between 1×10^{-4} and 8×10^{-4} M.
   - Prepare five 50 ml volumetric flasks (1 to 5). In each one, put the volume (ml) of solutions indicated in the table below. Add ferric chloride solution as shown in the table.

- Add distilled water to fill the flask to 50 ml.
- Swirl the flash to obtain homogeneous solutions.
- Measure the absorbance of the solutions (wavelength = 540 nm).
- Plot the calibration curve. absorbance vs. concentration (M).

	1	2	3	4	5
Salicylic acid (0.01 M)	0.5 ml	1 ml	2 ml	3 ml	4 ml
FeCl₃ (aq)	0.1 ml	0.2 ml	0.4 ml	0.6 ml	0.8 ml
Dilute to 50 ml exactly with distilled water					
C (mol/L)	1×10^{-4}	2×10^{-4}	4×10^{-4}	6×10^{-4}	8×10^{-4}
(salicylic acid concentration)					
Absorbance (540 nm)	0.198	0.404	0.586	0.784	0.982

2. **Preparation of the aspirin sample:** Place 0.2 g of aspirin into a 50 ml flask. Add ethanol (5 ml approximately) to dissolve it. Add a 1 ml solution of $FeCl_3$, and fill the flask upto mark (if a precipitate appears, add a little more ethanol and dilute after that to 50 ml). The observed color must be included in the calibration scale. If the observed color is too intense, dilute the solution.

3. **Determination of salicylic acid concentration in aspirin sample:** Measure the absorbance of the sample solution by means of the spectrophotometer. Use the calibration curve to calculate the concentration of the complexed salicylic acid (C) in the solution.

As shown in Fig. 15.4, the absorbance is 0.866 which corresponds to 0.000528 mole/L

$$C = 0.000528 \text{ mole/L or } 5.28 \times 10^{-4} \text{ mole/L}$$

Observation and calculation

% salicylic acid in aspirin:

$$\text{Salicylic acid } (\%) = \frac{5.28 \times 10^{-4} \times 138}{0.2} \times 100 = 36.4\%$$

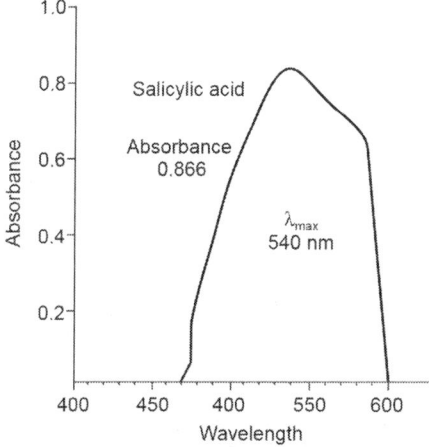

Fig. 15.4: Absorption spectrum of salicylic acid (sample).

Result

The amount of salicylic acid in aspirin is 36.4%.

Judge yourself

1. What is standard curve?
2. State Beer-Lambert law.
3. What is the reaction of ferric chloride and salicylic acid?
4. What do you mean by the term 'λ_{max}'?

EXPERIMENT 56

Determination of trimethoprim content in co-trimoxazole tablets

Co-trimoxazole tablets is a combination of trimethoprim (80 mg to 160 mg) and sulphamethoxazole (400 mg to 800 mg) and results in synergistic bactericidal effects. The action of co-trimoxazole is achieved by the sequential blocking of two enzymes essential in folinic acid synthesis in the organism. Sulfamethoxazole inhibits bacterial synthesis of dihydrofolic acid by competing with PABA. Trimethoprim blocks production of tetrahydrofolic acid by inhibiting the enzyme dihydrofolate reductase. This combination blocks 2 consecutive steps in bacterial biosynthesis of essential nucleic acids and proteins and is usually bactericidal.

Experimental overview

Sulfamethoxazole is determined by diazotiztion method due to presence of primary aromatic amino group (refer diazotization method).

Trimethoprim is determined by spectrophotometric method. Its shows the maximum absorption at 271 nm.

Trimethoprim

$$A = A_{1\ cm}^{1\%}.b.c$$

A = absorbance

$A_{1\ cm}^{1\%}$ = specific absorbance (204 nm)

b = path length (it is constant)

c = the concentration

Reagents required

1. 0.1 M NaOH solution.
2. Chloroform.
3. Dilute acetic acid.

Procedure

For trimethoprim

1. **Preparation of standard solution:** Weigh accurately about 0.05 g of trimethoprim (standard). Dissolve in sufficient 1.0 M acetic acid and make up the volume up to 250 ml with 1.0 M acetic acid. To the 10.0 ml of this add 1.0 M acetic acid to make up the 100 ml in volumetric flask.
2. **Preparation of unknown:**
   (i) Weigh and powder 20 tablets.
   (ii) Weigh accurately a quantity of powder equivalent to about 0.05 g of trimethoprim.

(iii) Add to it 30 ml of 0.1 M NaOH solution, mix, extract with four successive quantities, each of 50 ml of chloroform, washing each extract with same two quantities, each of 10 ml of 0.1 M NaOH solution.

(iv) Combine the chloroform extract and extract with four successive quantities, each of 50 ml of 1.0 M acetic acid. Wash the combined aqueous extract with 50 ml of chloroform and dilute the aqueous extract to 250.0 ml with 1.0 M acetic acid.

(v) To 10 ml of the solution, add 10 ml of 1.0 M acetic acid and sufficient water to produce 100.0 ml

(vi) Measure the absorbance of resulting solution and standard solution at about 271 nm against the blank prepared by diluting 10.0 ml of 1.0 M acetic acid to 100 ml with water.

Observation and calculation

For determination of trimethoprim

For example,

Average weight of tablet: 592.1 mg

Weight of tablet powder: 377.3 mg

Weight of trimethoprim powder (standard): 50.7 mg

Absorbance, tablet powder (A_{test}): 0.466

Absorbance, standard (A_{std}): 0.463

% purity of trimethoprim = 99%

$$\text{The content of trimethoprim per tablet} = \frac{T_{abs} \times \text{Std. wt.} \times \text{Potency of std.} \times \text{Av. wt.}}{\text{Std}_{abs} \times \text{Test wt.} \times 100} = \dots \text{mg}$$

$$\text{The content of trimethoprim per tablet} = \frac{0.466 \times 50.7 \times 99 \times 592.1}{0.463 \times 377.3 \times 100} = 79.3 \text{ mg}$$

where 99/100 is the percentage purity of trimethoprim

Note: The content of trimethoprim ($C_{14}H_{18}N_4O_6$) can be calculated by taking 204 the value of A (1%, 1 cm) at the λ max 271 nm (IP method)

For example, absorbance = 0.261.

Hence, concentration = 0.262/204 = g/100 ml.

But this type of method can only be followed when instrument is calibrated.

Judge yourself

1. How the sulfamethoxazole and trimethoprim show synergistic action? Explain.
2. What structural features are responsible for UV absorption in trimethoprim?
3. Why sodium hydroxide is added in the determination of trimethoprim?

EXPERIMENT 57

Spectrophotometric determination of metronidazole tablets

Reference

Journal of the Iranian Chemical Society, Vol. 2, No. 3, September 2005, pp. 197–202.

Experimental overview

5-Nitroimidazoles, such as metronidazole, are extensively used as anti-amoebic, anti-protozoal and antibacterial drugs.

Metronidazole is officially determined by titrimetry, potentiometry and HPLC methods. Indian Pharmacopoeia describes the non-aqueous titration method using perchloric acid as titrant and malachite green as indicator for the assay of metronidazole. British Pharmacopoeia describes potentiometric and non-aqueous titration methods using perchloric acid as titrant. United States Pharmacopoeia describes HPLC and nonaqueous titration methods for the assay of metronidazole. Visible spectrophotometry, because of simplicity and cost effectiveness, sensitivity and selectivity, and fair accuracy and precision, has remained competitive for its determination. Most of the spectrophotometric methods found in the literature for the determination of metronidazole in the visible region involve initial reduction by treatment with Zinc powder and HCl followed by the diazotization and coupling of the resulting amine.

Metronidazole   Metronidazole (reduced form)

R = CH_2CH_2OH (Complex)

The present spectrophotometric method for the determination of metronidazole is based on the reduction of the nitro group to amino group of the drug. This can be achieved by heating a mixture of an alcoholic solution of metronidazole, zinc powder and dilute hydrochloric acid in a water bath at 90 ± 5°C for 15 min. The cold and clear filtrate reacts with *p*-benzoquinone to develop a purple color, which absorbs maximally at 526 nm. The calibration graph is linear over the concentration range of 15–190 µg ml^{-1}. This method can be applied to commercially available pharmaceutical dosage forms.

Reagents required

1. Zinc powder.

2. *p*-Benzoquinone solution. Dissolve 8 mg of *p*-benzoquinone in a minimum amount of ethanol in a 100 ml volumetric flask and make up the volume with ethanol.
3. 5 N HCl solution.

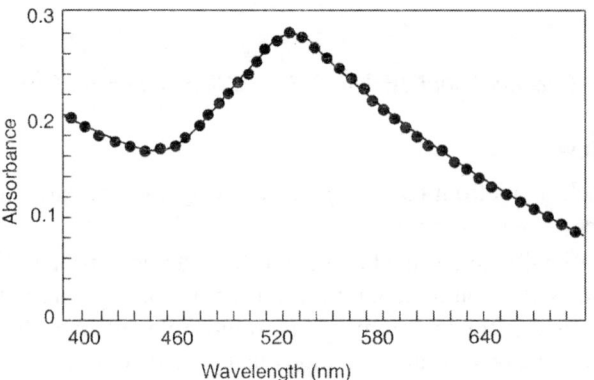

Fig. 15.5: Absorption spectrum of metronidazole.

Procedure

A. **Reduced metronidazole standard stock solution:** Dissolve 79 mg of metronidazole in 30 ml hot ethanol and add to it 5 ml of 5 N HCl solution and 1 mg of zinc dust. Heat the mixture on a water bath at $90 \pm 5°C$ for 15 min. Cool, filter and then wash with ethanol. Make up the volume to 100 ml with ethanol in a volumetric flask to obtain the standard solution with a concentration of 790 µg ml^{-1}.

B. **Construction of calibration curve:** Into a series of twelve 50 ml volumetric flasks, take reduced metronidazole standard stock solution equivalent to 15–190 µg ml^{-1} (1 to 12 ml). Add to each flask 1 ml of *p*-benzoquinone solution and bring the volume up to 50 ml with ethanol. Measure the absorbance at 526 nm against a reagent blank. Construct the calibration curve by plotting the absorbance against the concentration.

C. **Determination of metronidazole tablets:** Weigh accurately 20 tablets of metronidazole and powder them. Calculate the average weight of tablet. Weigh accurately quantity of powder equivalent to 100–400 mg of metronidazole. Carry out the reduction of metronidazole as mentioned above. Transfer the resulting filtrate to a 100 ml volumetric flask and make up to the mark with ethanol. Treat 1 ml of this reduced metronidazole with 1 ml of *p*-benzoquinone and make up the volume to 50 ml with ethanol in a volumetric flask. Measure the absorbance of this solution.

Observation and calculation

Average weight of metronidazole tablet: W g

Weight of tablet powder: W_1 g

Plot a calibration curve as shown in Fig. 15.6.

Read out the concentration of metronidazole from calibration curve. Multiply with the dilution factor to get the final concentration.

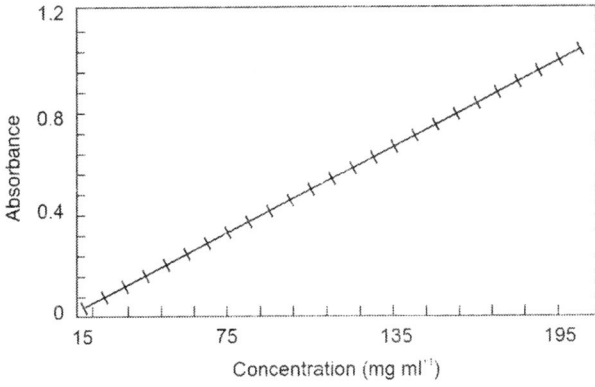

Fig. 15.6: Calibration curve of metronidazole.

Judge yourself

1. How metronidazole acts as anti-amoebic agent?

2. Mention the various types of reducing agents which can be applied for the reduction of nitro group in metronidazole.

3. What happen if metronidazole after reduction followed by diazotization is subjected to a condensation reaction with aromatic aldehyde namely, vanillin and p-dimethyl amino benzaldehyde (PDAB)? Predict the λ_{max} of resulting product.

EXPERIMENT 58

Determination of ranitidine content in tablets

Experimental overview

Ranitidine hydrochloride (RNH), chemically is N,N-dimethyl-5-[2-(1-methylamine-2–nitrovinyl)-ethylthiomethyl] furfurylamine hydrochloride. It is a H_2-receptor antagonist and is widely used in short term treatment of duodenal ulcer and in the management of hypersecretory conditions.

$$(CH_3)_2N-CH_2 \underset{O}{\diagup\diagdown} -CH_2-S-(CH_2)_2-NH\diagdown \atop H_3C-HN \diagup C=CH-NO_2$$

Ranitidine

The tablet contains contain 150 or 300 mg of ranitidine base. It absorbs at the wavelength 313 nm in the visible region. This wavelength is utilized for its spectrometric determination.

Reagents required

1. Ranitidine HCl (standard).
2. Distilled water.

Procedure

1. **Preparation of standard ranitidine HCl solution:**
   (i) Weigh accurately 100 mg of ranitidine HCl.
   (ii) Dissolve in sufficient distilled water and make up the volume to 100 ml in volumetric flask.
   (iii) Pipet out 2 ml of this solution in 100 ml volumetric flask and make up the volume.
   (iv) Measure the absorbance at 313 nm (λ_{max}).

2. **Preparation of unknown ranitidine HCl solution:**
   (i) Weigh accurately 20 tablets. Find out the average weight of tablet.
   (ii) Powder them and weigh accurately the powder equivalent to 100 mg of ranitidine HCl. Dissolve in a sufficient distilled water and make up the volume to 100 ml in a volumetric flask.
   (iii) Pipet out 2 ml of this solution in 100 ml volumetric flask and make up the volume.
   (iv) Measure the absorbance at 313 nm (λ_{max}).

Observation and calculation

Average weight of tablet: W_1 g

Weight of powder equivalent to 100 mg of ranitidine HCl: W_2 g

Weight of ranitidine HCl (standard): W_3 g

Absorbance of ranitidine HCl (standard): A_{St}

Absorbance of ranitidine HCl (tablet): A_{Test}

% purity of ranitidine: 99%

The content of ranitidine (base) in tablet $= \dfrac{A_{\text{Test}} \times W_3 \times 314.37 \times 99}{A_{\text{St}} \times W_2 \times 350.87 \times 100} \times W_1 = \ldots\, \text{g}$

Note: Dilution factor is same in standard and test solution. Hence, it is taken as 1. 314.37 and 350.87 are the molecular weight of ranitidine base and ranitidine HCl respectively.

Result

The content of ranitidine (base) in tablet : .... g

Alternate method

The tablet can also be assayed by making the calibration curve. For this, make the stock solution of ranitidine HCl containing 1 mg/ml. Then make further dilution of ranitidine HCl solution containing 0.1 to 20 µg. Measure the absorbance. Make a calibration curve by plotting a graph between concentration and absorbance. Then, make the same dilution from the tablet in this concentration range. Measure the absorbance and read out the concentration from the calibration curve.

Judge yourself

1. How ranitidine acts as antiulcer drug?
2. Which moiety in ranitidine is responsible for absorption in UV region?
3. Show the calculation of ranitidine base if dilution is different.

EXPERIMENT 59

Determination of paracetamol content in tablet

METHOD I

Experimental overview

Paracetamol is a widely used over-the-counter analgesic (pain reliever) and antipyretic (fever reducer). It is commonly used for the relief of fever, headaches, and other minor aches and pains, and is a major ingredient in numerous cold and flu remedies. In combination with non-steroidal anti-inflammatory drugs (NSAIDs) or opioid analgesics, paracetamol is used also in the management of more severe pain (such as cancer pain).

It shows three λ_{max} at 242, 243 and 257 nm in neutral, acidic and alkaline media respectively. The present experiment is a estimation of paracetamol in alkaline media. Paracetamol shows maximum absorption at 257 nm due to presence of phenyl ring in alkaline media. The absorbance of different dilution of paracetamol is taken at this wavelength to make the calibration curve. The absorbance of unknown sample is taken and with the help of calibration curve, the concentration is read out.

| Paracetamol | | Sodium salt of paracetamol |

Reagents required

1. Paracetamol reference substance.
2. NaOH.

Procedure

(i) Accurately weigh 100 mg of paracetamol reference substance into a 100 ml volumetric flask, dissolve with 50 ml of 0.1 M NaOH solution. Dilute to volume with water, mix well.

(ii) Separately transfer accurately 0.1, 0.2 .... to 1 ml of this solution into 10 different 10 ml volumetric flask and dilute with 0.1 M NaOH solution to the mark. The concentration range is 0.32~1.92 mg/ml.

(iii) Measure the absorbance of the each solution at 257 nm.

(iv) Weigh accurately and powder finely 10 tablets, weigh accurately a portion of the powder (equivalent to about 100 mg of paracetamol) into 100 ml volumetric flask, add 50 ml of 0.1 M NaOH solution, mix for 15 minutes.

(v) Filter if necessary. Make up the volume with 0.1 M NaOH solution.

(vi) Transfer 0.5 ml of this solution and dilute to 10 ml in volumetric flask.

Observation and calculation

Absorbance value of paracetamol

S. No.	Concentration	Absorbance
1.	–	
2.	–	
3.	–	
4.	–	
5.	–	
6.	–	
Unknown	–	

Plot a calibration curve by plotting a graph between absorbance of different standard dilution and their concentration. Read out a concentration of unknown from calibration curve. Multiply the concentration with dilution factor to find out the initial concentration.

Note: Calculation can also be done by considering specific absorbance of paracetamol, 715, as specified in IP.

$$A = a.b.c$$

$$C = \frac{\text{Absorbance of unknown}}{715}$$

METHOD II

Reference: Analyst 111, 919–921 (1986).

Experimental view

Cerium (IV) sulphate is heated for 90 minutes with paracetamol in concentrated sulfuric acid in waterbath maintained at 80°C. The final product of oxidation, *p*-benzoquinone is determined spectrophoto-metrically at the wavelength of its maximum absorption, 410 nm.

The calibration curve is plotted using different concentration of standard paracetamol. Then, absorbance value of unknown solution is measured. From the calibration curve, the concentration of unknown solution/tablet is read out. Beer's law is valid over the concentration range between 30 and 160 mg/ml.

Reagents required

1. Paracetamol reference substance
2. 10 M sulfuric acid solution
3. Cerium (IV) sulphate solution. Prepare a stock solution of Ce $(SO_4)_2$ (20 mg/ml) in 10 M Sulfuric acid.

Procedure

(i) Prepare the stock solution of paracetamol (1 mg/ml) by dissolving 1.0 g in sufficient warm water. Stir for 10 minutes and make up the volume 1 litre in volumetric flask.

(ii) Dilute 1 ml of this solution to 100 ml with water in volumetric flask.

(iii) Weigh accurately 20 tablets of paracetamol and ground them into a fine powder. Weigh accurately about 500 mg of paracetamol, mix with about 150 ml of water, warm and stir for 10 minutes Filter, wash the filter paper with sufficient water and make up the volume to 500 ml in a volumetric flask.

(iv) Dilute 1 ml of this solution to 10 ml with water.

(v) Place a 4.00 ml volume of cerium (IV) sulfate solution in a 50 ml calibrated flask to which add 21.00 ml of sulfuric acid and the appropriate amount (1 ml) of paracetamol solution. Swirl the flask and contents, place in a water-bath at a temperature maintained at 80°C for 90 min, cool under a tap and then dilute to the mark with water. Determine the absorbance at 410 nm against a reagent blank.

(vi) Similarly, do the same with unknown sample (tablet).

Observation and calculation

Sample calculation

Average weight of tablet: P g

Weight of tablet powder equivalent to 0.5 g of paracetamol: W g

Weight of paraetamol powder (standard): 0.8 g/litre

Absorbance, tablet powder: A_{Test}

Absorbance, standard: A_{Abs}

$$\text{Content of paracetamol per tablet} = \frac{T_{(abs)} \times \text{Std wt} \times \% \text{ purity of std.} \times \text{Av. wt.}}{\text{Std}_{(abs)} \times \text{Test wt} \times 100} = ... \text{ mg}$$

Judge yourself

1. How % purity of paracetamol can be determined?
2. Mention the reaction of paracetamol and ceric sulfate.
3. What is molar absorptivity?

EXPERIMENT 60

Determination of amoxycilln content in capsule

Experimental overview

Amoxycillin is a moderate spectrum, β-lactam antibiotic used to treat bacterial infections caused by susceptible microorganism.

The capsule contains 250 or 500 mg of $C_{16}H_{19}N_3O_5S$, calculated with reference to anhydrous base. Its structure is:

Reagents required

1. Amoxycillin reference substance.
2. *p*-Dimethylaminobenzaldehyde (PDAB). Dissolve 0.4 g of PDAB in 10 ml of alcohol. Add to it 2 ml of conc. Sulfuric acid solution. Make up the volume to 50 ml with water.
3. Alcohol.

Procedure

1. **Preparation of standard amoxicillin solution:** Weigh accurately about 150 mg of amoxicillin and dissolve in sufficient distilled water and make up the volume to 100 ml volumetric flask. It is the stock solution containing 1.5 mg/ml of amoxicillin. From this solution, take 0.1 to 10 ml in 10 different flask and make up the volume to 10 ml. From above standard, pipet out 2 ml and add 4 ml of PDAB. Heat for 1 hr on a waterbath. Cool down and make up the volume to 10 ml with distilled water in volumetric flask.
2. **Preparation of test sample solution:**
   (i) Weigh accurately 20 capsule and find out the average weight of capsule.
   (ii) Weigh accurately powder equivalent to 150 mg of amoxicillin. Dissolve in sufficient distilled water and make up the volume to 100 ml.
   (iii) Take 1 ml of this solution and dilute up to 10 ml with distilled water in volumetric flask.
   (iv) Pipet out 2 ml of amoxicillin, add 4 ml of PDAB and heat on water bath for 1 hr. Cool down and make up the volume to 10 ml.
3. Measure the absorbance of each standard and test sample at 410 nm.

Observation and calculation

Average weight of capsule: W_1 g
Average weight of capsule powder equivalent to 150 mg of amoxicillin: W_2 g
Plot a calibration curve by plotting a graph between concentration (mg) and absorbance. Read out the concentration of Test solution from the calibration curve.

Suppose, it is 36.5 g.

The amount of amoxycillin in the sample = 36.5 × 100 × 10 × 5 = 91.5 mg where 100 × 10 × 5 is the dilution factor.

Table 15.2: Absorbance of amoxycillin solution

S. No.	Final concentration of Amoxycillin (μg/10 ml)	Absorbance
1.	30	–
2.	60	–
3.	90	–
4.	120	–
5.	150	–
6.	180	–
7.	210	–
8.	240	–
9.	270	–
10.	300	–
11.	Unknown	–

W_2 g test sample contain = 91.5 mg of amoxycillin

Amount of amoxycillin present in average weight capsule $= \dfrac{91.5 \times W_1}{W_2} = $ g

Alternate method

Take the absorbance of amoxycillin reference substance and test sample (capsule) after preparing the standard and test sample in the same concentration range.

Average weight of capsule: W_1 g

Weight of powder equivalent to 150 mg of amoxycillin: W_2 g

Weight of amoxycillin HCl (standard): W_3 g

Absorbance of amoxycillin (standard): A_{St}

Absorbance of amoxycillin (capsule): A_{Test}

The content of amoxycillin (anhydrous base) usually present = 85%

Note: Amoxycillin trihydrate contains about 14.5% moisture

Content of amoxycillin (base) in capsule $= \dfrac{A_{Test} \times W_3 \times 85 \times 371.48}{A_{St} \times W_2 \times 100 \times 419.45} = W_1 = ...$ g amoxycillin

where 371.48 and 419.45 are the molecular weight of amoxycillin base and amoxycillin trihydrate respectively.

Note: Keep the same dilution factor in standard and test solution so that it is taken as 1. Otherwise mention the dilution factor in the calculation.

Result

The content of amoxycillin (base) in capsule: .... g.

Judge yourself

1. What is the reaction of PDAB with amoxycillin?
2. Mention the significance of calibration curve.
3. What are the uses of amoxycillin trihydrate?

EXPERIMENT 61

Determination of tadalafil content in tablet

Experimental overview

Tadalafil is an orally administered drug for treating erectile dysfunction (ED). Moreover, besides ED, tadalafil for the treatment of pulmonary arterial hypertension is currently under regulatory review in multiple regions. It act by inhibition of phosphodiesterase type 5 (PDE5) which enhances erectile function by increasing the amount of cGMP.

Tadalafil

It absorbs at 292 nm (UV region) so Beer-lambert law can be utilized for its estimation.

Reagents required

1. Tadalafil reference substance.
2. Methanol.

Procedure

1. **Preparation of standard tadalafil solution:** Weigh accurately about 50 mg of tadalafil in 50 ml volumetric flask and dissolve in sufficient methanol and make up the volume with methanol. Pipet out 2 ml of this solution and dilute up to 100 ml with methanol in 100 ml volumetric flask. It is stock solution containing 20 mg/ml of tadalafil.
2. **Preparation of test sample:** Weigh accurately 20 tablets and powder them. Weigh accurately powder equivalent to 50 mg of tadalafil and transfer into 50 ml volumetric flask. Pipet out 2 ml of this solution and dilute up to 100 ml with methanol in 100 ml volumetric flask.
3. Take the absorbance of standard solution and test sample at 292 nm (λ_{max}) by taking methanol as blank solution.

Observation and calculation

Average weight of tablet: W_1 g

Weight of powder equivalent to 50 mg of tadalafil: W_2 g

Weight of tadalafil (standard): W_3 g

Absorbance of tadalafil (standard): A_{St}

Absorbance of tadalafil (tablet): A_{Test}

% purity of tadalafil : 99%

The content of tadalafil in tablet $= \dfrac{A_{Test} \times W_3 \times 99 \times W_1}{A_{St} \times W_2 \times 100} = \ldots$ g tadalafil

Note: Dilution factor in standard and test solution is same. Hence, it is taken as 1. Otherwise mention the dilution factor in the calculation.

Result

The content of tadalafil in tablet: .... g.

Judge yourself

1. How tadalafil acts?
2. What is moiety responsible for absorption in UV region in tadalafil?
3. Name the other drugs which are phosphodientrase type V inhibitors.

EXPERIMENT 62

Spectrophotometric determination of chloroquine phosphate content in tablet

Chloroquine (7-chloro-4-(4-diethylamino-1-methylbutylamino)quinoline;possesses an asymmetric carbon atom and therefore exists as two enantiomers, S (+)–chloroquine and R(–)–chloroquine.Its structure is shown below. Only preparations containing the racemic mixture are commercially available.

Chloroquine phosphate is freely soluble in water. An aqueous solubility of 1 in 4 was reported. It is not clear if this means 1 part dissolved in 4 part solution, i.e., 250 mg/ml, or 1 part dissolvable in 4 parts of water, i.e., 200 mg/ml.

Chloroquine is used in the treatment and prophylaxis of malaria and has also been used in the treatment of hepatic amoebiasis, lupus erythematosus, and light-sensitive skin eruptions. Chloroquine possesses antiinflammatory properties and rheumatoid arthritis is a further indication for this drug.

Experimental overview

Chloroquine phosphate is analyzed spectrophotometrically at the wavelength of 343 nm, using water as blank.

Reagents required

1. Chloroquine phosphate reference.
2. Distilled water.

Procedure

1. Weigh accurately about 0.250 g of chloroquine phosphate reference and dissolve in 200 ml of water by shaking. Adjust the volume to 250 ml. Dilute 10 ml of this solution to 100 ml in volumetric flask.
2. Weigh accurately 20 tablets and find out the average weight.
3. Weigh accurately the powder equivalent to 0.250 g of chloroquine phosphate and dissolve in about 200 ml of water by mechanical shaking for 30 minutes. Adjust the volume to 250 ml.
4. Filter, reject the first 25 ml and dilute 10 ml of this solution to 100 ml in volumetric flask.
5. Measure the absorbance of both the solution at 343 nm.

Observation and calculation

Average weight of chloroquine phosphate tablet: W_1 g

Weight of powder equivalent to 0.250 g of chloroquine phosphate: W_2 g

Weight of chloroquine phosphate (standard): W_3 g

Absorbance of chloroquine phosphate (standard): A_{St}

Absorbance of chloroquine phosphate (tablet): A_{Test}

% purity of chloroquine phosphate: 99%

Content of chloroquine phosphate/tablet $= \dfrac{A_{Test} \times W_3 \times 99 \times W_1}{A_{St} \times W_2 \times 100} = ...$ g chloroquine phosphate.

Note: Dilution factor in standard and test solution is same. Hence, it is taken as 1. Otherwise mention the dilution factor in the calculation.

$$\% \text{ content} = \frac{\text{Content / tablet}}{\text{Declared strength}} \times 100 = ... \%$$

Result

The content of chloroquine phosphate in tablet: .... g

Judge yourself

1. How chloroquine acts?
2. What is moiety responsible for absorption in UV region in chloroquine?
3. How λ_{max} is determined?

EXPERIMENT 63

UV spectrophotometric methods for simultaneous estimation of ibuprofen and paracetamol in tablet by simultaneous equation method

Ibuprofen [RS-2-(4-isobutyl-phenyl) propionic acid], is one of the most potent orally active anti-pyretic, analgesic and non steroidal anti-inflammatory drug (NSAID) used extensively in the treatment of acute and chronic pain, osteoarthritis, rheumatoid arthritis and related conditions. This compound is characterized by a better tolerability compared with other NSAIDs.

Paracetamol is 4'-hydroxyacetanilide. It is antipyretic and analgesic.

Procedure

Procedure for calibration curve:

1. Weigh accurately 10 mg of ibuprofen (IBU) standard solutions and dissolve in water and make up the volume to 100 ml in volumetric flask (100 mcg/ml). It will be a stock solution.
2. Prepare the different dilution of ibuprofen in the concentration range of 4 µg/ml to 14 µg/ml obtained by transferring (0.4, 0.6, 0.8, 1.0, 1.2, 1.4 ml) of ibuprofen stock solution (100 µg/ml) to the series of 10 ml volumetric flasks.
3. Similarly, prepare the stock solution of paracetamol (PCM) and different dilutions of standard solutions of paracetamol in the concentration range of 2 µg/ml to 12 µg/ml by transferring (0.2, 0.4, 0.6, 0.8, 1.0, 1.2 ml) of PCM stock solution (100 µg/ml) to the series of 10 ml volumetric flasks.
4. Add methanol to each volumetric flask up to 10 ml.
5. Scan any one dilution (e.g. 10 µg/ml) for each drug in wavelength range of 200 nm to 400 nm to know their λ_{max}.

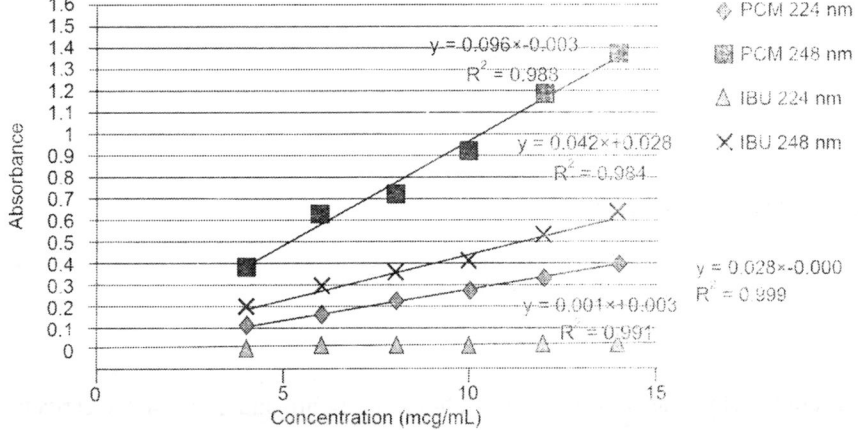

Fig. 15.7: Calibration curves of PCM and IBU.

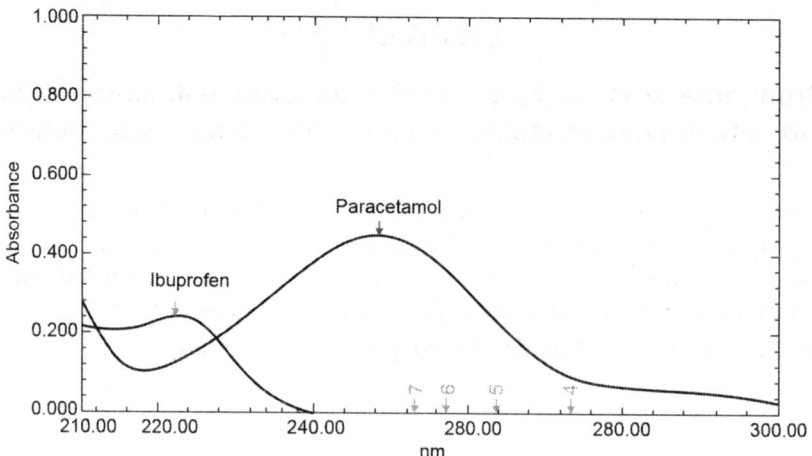

Fig. 15.8. Overlay spectra of ibuprofen and paracetamol.

6. Take absorbances of all prepared dilutions of both drugs (PCM and IBU) at their respective identified λ_{max}.
7. The absorbances were plotted against the respective concentrations to obtain the calibration curves (Fig. 15.6).
8. A representative overlay spectrum of IBU and PCM in methanol is shown in Fig. 15.7.

Estimation of ibuprofen and paracetamol in tablet dosage form

1. Weigh accurately of 20 tablets and calculate the average content weight of one capsule.
2. Take average content weight of one tablet. Add 80 ml of methanol; heat it for 25 minutes at 50–55°C.
3. Filter this solution and make up the volume of filtrate with methanol up to 100 ml, i.e. it contains 400 mg/100 ml of IBU and 325 mg/100 ml of PCM. One ml of this solution contains 4 mg and 3.25 mg of PCM and IBU respectively.
4. Dilute this solution appropriately to get approximate concentration of 6 µg/ml of IBU and 5 µg/ml of PCM.
   Note: Dilute 1.0 ml of the above solution to 100 ml to get concentration of 40 mcg/ml and 32.5 mcg/ml IBU and PCM respectively. Dilute 1.5 ml of this solution 10 ml to get the concentration of 6 mcg/ml and 4.875 mcg/ml of IBU and PCM respectively.
5. Measure the absorbance of sample solution at 224 nm and 248 nm against blank.
6. Calculate the content of IBU and PCM in solution (mcg) using two framed simultaneous equations.
7. Finally, calculate the content in tablet using dilution factor.

Formation of simultaneous equation

Set of two simultaneous equations are:

$C_x = (A_2 ay_1 - A_1 ay_2)/ (ax_2 ay_1 - ax_1 ay_2)$ and
$C_y = (A_1 ax_2 - A_2 ax_1)/ (ax_2 ay_1 - ax_1 ay_2)$,

where

A_1 and A_2 are the absorbance of sample solutions at 224 nm and 248 nm respectively.
C_x and C_y are concentrations of IBU and PCM in mg/ml in sample solution.

By substituting the values of A_1 and A_2 the values of C_x and C_y can be calculated by solving the two equations simultaneously.

Here, ax_1 and ax_2 are the absorptivity coefficient of IBU at 224 nm and 248 nm respectively; ay_1 and ay_2 are the absorptivity coefficient of PCM at 224 nm and 248 nm, respectively.

To get absorptivity divide the absorbance by path lengh and concentration

$$\varepsilon = A/lc$$

where A is the amount of light absorbed by the sample for a given wavelength, ε is the molar absorptivity, l is the distance that the light travels through the solution, and c is the concentration of the absorbing species per unit volume.

Standard units for molar absorptivity are litres per mole centimeter (L mol^{-1} cm^{-1})

The linearity range for IBU and PCM were 4–14 µg/ml and 2–12 µg/ ml, respectively.

Observation and calculation

Absorptivity of paracetamol at λ 248 nm (ax_1) = 0.0968

Absorbtivity of paracetamol at λ 224 nm (ay_1) = 0.0284

Absorbtivity of Ibuprofen at λ 248 nm (ax_2) = 0.042

Absorbtivity of Ibuprofen at λ 224 nm (ay_2) = 0.0013

Absorbance of mixture (paracetamol + ibuprofen) at λ 248 nm (A_1) = 0.241

Absorbance of mixture (paracetamol + ibuprofen) at λ 224 nm (A_2) = 0.170

Paracetamol $C_x = (A_2ay_1 - A_1ay_2)/ (ax_2ay_1 - ax_1ay_2)$

$\qquad = 0.10 \times 0.0284 - 0.241 \times 0.0013/0.042 \times 0.0284 - 0.0968 \times 0.0013$

$\qquad = 4.76$ mcg/ml

Ibupofen $C_y = (A_1ax_2 - A_2ax_1)/ (ax_2ay_1 - ax_1ay_2)$

$\qquad = 0.241 \times 0.042 - 0.17 \times 0.0968/0.042 \times 0.0284 - 0.0968 \times 0.0013$

$\qquad = 5.9$ mcg/ml

Result

Calibration curve data of paracetamol and ibuprofen

Conc. (mcg/ml)	PCM (224 nm)	PCM (248 nm)	IBU (224 nm)	IBU (248 nm)
4	0.117	0.385	0.009	0.204
6	0.167	0.628	0.011	0.296
8	0.225	0.724	0.013	0.353
10	0.282	0.918	0.016	0.416
12	0.34	1.081	0.019	0.529
14	0.4	1.37	0.022	0.639

	Drug concentration in diluted sample (mcg/ml)	Drug claims in tablet (mg)	Drug concentration found in diluted sample (mcg/ml)	Drug found (mg)
PCM	4.875	325	4.76	317.3
IBU	6.0	400	5.9	393.3

High Performance Liquid Chromatography (HPLC)

Introduction

High Performance Liquid Chromatography (HPLC) is mode of chromatography, the most widely used analytical technique. HPLC utilizes a liquid mobile phase to separate the components of a mixture. These components (or analytes) are first dissolved in a solvent, and then forced to flow through a chromatographic column under a high pressure. In the column, the mixture is resolved into its components.

The interaction of the solute with mobile and stationary phases can be manipulated through different choices of both solvents and stationary phases. As a result, HPLC acquires a high degree of versatility not found in other chromatographic systems and it has the ability to easily separate a wide variety of chemical mixtures.

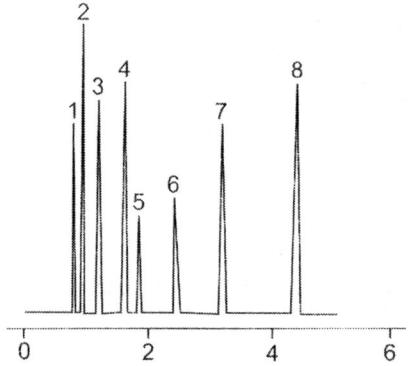

Fig. 16.1. Fast and high-efficient separation of some aromatics. Hypersil-C8 (100 × 2) 3 mm, 60% MeOH in water, 1.5 ml min., 1 - Benzamide, 2 - Benzyl alcohol, 3 - Acetophenone, 4 - Methyl benzoate, 5 - Phenetole, 6 - Naphthalene, 7 - Benzophenone, 8 - Biphenyl.

Types of HPLC

There are many ways to classify liquid column chromatography. If this classification is based on the nature of the stationary phase and the separation process, three modes can be specified.

In adsorption chromatography the stationary phase is an adsorbent (like silica gel or any other silica based packings) and the separation is based on repeated adsorption-desorption steps.

In ion-exchange chromatography the stationary bed has an ionically charged surface of opposite charge to the sample ions. This technique is used almost exclusively with ionic or ionizable samples. The stronger the charge on the sample, the stronger it will be attracted to the ionic surface and thus, the longer it will take to elute. The mobile phase is an aqueous buffer, where both pH and ionic strength are used to control elution time.

In size exclusion chromatography the column is filled with material having precisely controlled pore sizes, and the sample is simply screened or filtered according to its solvated molecular size. Larger molecules are rapidly washed through the column; smaller molecules penetrate inside the porous of the packing particles and elute later. Mainly for historical reasons, this technique is also called gel filtration or gel permeation chromatography although, today, the stationary phase is not restricted to a "gel".

Concerning the first type, two modes are defined depending on the relative polarity of the two phases: **normal** and **reversed-phase chromatography.**

In normal-phase chromatography, the stationary bed is strongly polar in nature (e.g. silica gel), and the mobile phase is nonpolar (such as n-hexane or tetrahydrofuran). Polar samples are thus retained on the polar surface of the column packing longer than less polar materials.

Reversed-phase chromatography is the inverse of this. The stationary bed is nonpolar (hydrophobic) in nature, while the mobile phase is a polar liquid, such as mixtures of water and methanol or acetonitrile. Here the more nonpolar the material is, the longer it will be retained.

There are two elution types: isocratic and gradient.

In the first type constant eluent composition is pumped through the column during the whole analysis.

In the second type, eluent composition (and strength) is steadily changed during the run.

HPLC as compared with the classical technique is characterized by:

- Small diameter (2–5 mm), reusable stainless steel columns.
- Column packings with very small (3, 5 and 10 μm) particles.
- Relatively high inlet pressures and controlled flow of the mobile phase.
- Precise sample introduction without the need for large samples.
- Special continuous flow detectors capable of handling small flow rates and detecting very small amounts.
- Automated standardized instruments.
- Rapid analysis.
- High resolution.

Initially, pressure was selected as the principal criterion of modern liquid chromatography and thus the name was "high pressure liquid chromatography" or HPLC.

High performance is the result of many factors:

- Very small particles of narrow distribution range and uniform pore size and distribution.
- High pressure column slurry packing techniques.

- Accurate low volume sample injectors.
- Sensitive low volume detectors.
- Good pumping systems.

Pressure is needed to permit a given flow rate of the mobile phase; otherwise, pressure is a negative factor not contributing to the improvement in separation.

Recognizing this, most experienced chromatographers today, refer to the technique as high performance liquid chromatography still permitting the use of the acronym HPLC.

EXPERIMENT 64

HPLC determination of ranitidine HCl tablet

Ranitidine HCl is a H_2 receptor antagonist. It occurs as a white to pale-yellow granular substance with a bitter taste and a sulfur-like odor. The drug has pKas of 8.2 and 2.7. One gram is approximately soluble in 1.5 ml of water or 6 ml of alcohol. Ranitidine HCl tablets contains 75 mg or 150 mg or. 300 mg of ranitidine base).

$$(CH_3)_2NCH_2 \underset{O}{\overset{}{\bigcirc}} CH-S-CH_2CH_2CH_2NH-\underset{\underset{CHNO_2}{\|}}{C}-NHCH_3$$

Ranitidine

Experimental overview

The objective of this experiment is to determine the % of ranitidine base in ranitidie HCl tablet.

The instrument used in this experiment is a Simazdu LC system, consisting of LC-10ATVP pump and SPD-10AVP detector system.

Procedure

HPLC conditions:

Column: C_{18} 250 × 4.6 mm (5 mm).

Mobile phase: 85 volume of methanol and 15 volume of 0.1 M ammonium acetate.

Flow rate: 2.0 ml/min.

Injection volume: 20 µl.

Wavelength: 322 nm.

(A) **Preparation of solutions:**

  (1) *Stock:* Completely dissolve approximately 112 mg of ranitidine HCl in 100 ml of mobile phase.

  (2) *Standard solution:* Dilute 10 ml of stock solution to 100 ml with mobile phase in volumetric flask.

  (3) *Test sample:* Weigh and powder 20 tablets. Dissolve about 195 mg of powder with 50 ml of mobile phase, filter and dilute to 100 ml with mobile phase in volumetric flask. Dilute 10 ml of this solution to 100 ml with mobile phase.

(B) **Analysis:**

  (1) Inject the 20 microlitre of standard solution in the HPLC system and run the system following instructor's directions.

  (2) Print a chromatogram and integration information for each sample.

  (3) Similarly, do the same with test sample.

  Note: Sample chromatograms of standard and test are enclosed here for reference.

Observation and calculation

  Mass of ranitidine HCl (standard): 112.9 mg

  Average weight of tablet: 290 mg

Weight of powder dissolved in mobile phase: 195.6 mg

Concentration of ranitidine HCl in stock solution: 1.129 mg/ml

Concentration of ranitidine HCl in the standard solutions: 0.01 mg/ml

Molecular weight of ranitidine HCl = 350.87

Molecular weight of ranitidine base = 314.37

% purity of ranitidine HCl = 99%

Ranitidine HCl retention time: 7.15

Ranitidine HCl peak area (in standard): 20536.7540

Ranitidine HCl peak area (in test): 20470.0539

Dilution factor of standard and sample is same.

Calculation based on peak area analysis:

The content of ranitidine base equivalent to ranitidine HCl:

$$= \frac{20470.05 \times 112.9 \times 314.37}{20536.75 \times 195.6 \times 350.87} \times \frac{99}{100} \times 290 = 147.99 \text{ mg (claim 150 mg)}$$

Result

The average weight tablet contains 147.99 mg of ranitidine base.

Judge yourself

1. Which solvent mixture is normally used in HPLC?
2. How AR reagents differ from HPLC grade?
3. Compare the gas chromatography and HPLC.

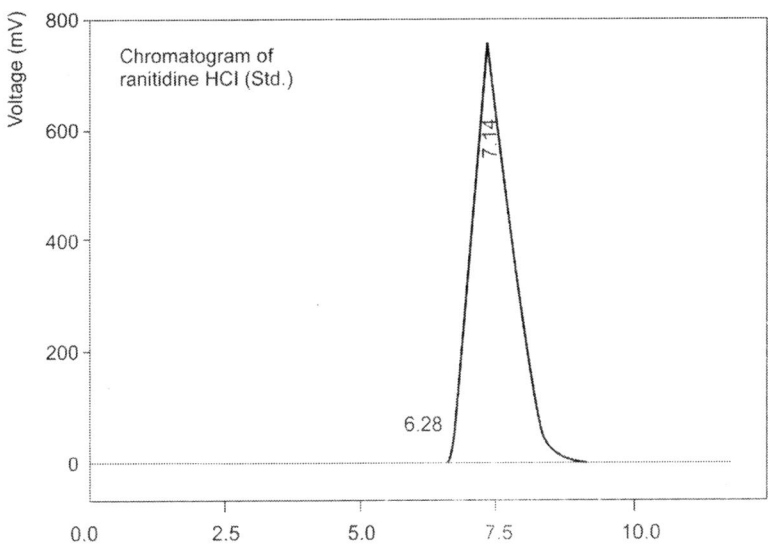

Result

Calculation method Uncal

Peak No.	Reten. time	Area [mV.s]	Height [mV]	W05 [min.]	Area [%]	Height [%]
1	6.280	26.8745	1.5955	0.3300	0.1307	0.2077
2	7.140	20536.7540	766.4566	0.3600	99.8693	99.7923
	Total	20563.6285	768.0521			

Column performance test report

Peak No.	Reten. time	W05 [min.]	Asymmetry [–]	Capacity [–]	Efficiency [th. pl.]	Eff./1 [t.p./m]	Resolution [–]	Ret. index [–]
1	6.280	0.330	0.864	5.28	2008	20081	–	
2	7.140	0.360	1.774	6.14	2181	21812	1.567	0

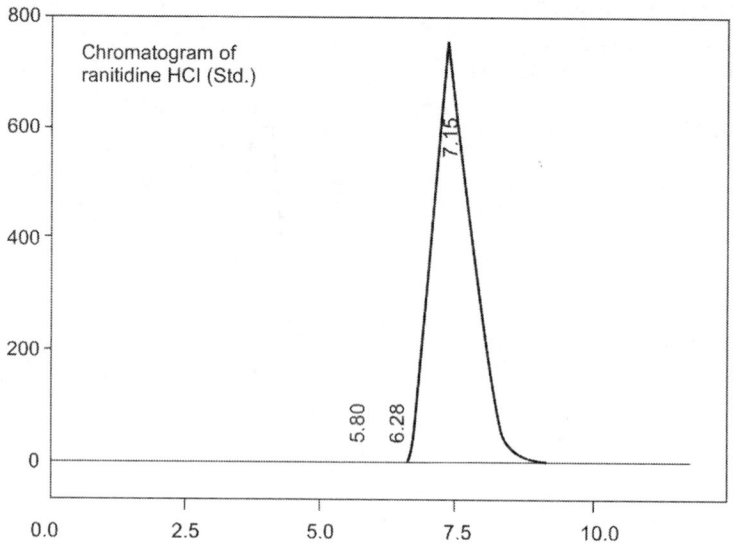

Result

Calculation method Uncal

Peak No.	Reten. time	Area [mV.s]	Height [mV]	W05 [min.]	Area [%]	Height [%]
1	5.800	2.1325	0.1903	0.2200	0.0104	0.0243
2	6.280	29.9594	1.7547	0.3400	0.1461	0.2240
3	7.150	20470.0539	781.3479	0.3600	99.8435	99.7517
	Total	20502.1458	783.2929			

Column performance test report

Peak No.	Reten. time	W05 [min.]	Asymmetry [–]	Capacity [–]	Efficiency [th. pl.]	Eff./1 [t.p./m]	Resolution [–]	Ret. index [–]
1	5.800	0.220	0.938	0.480	3854	38540	–	0
2	6.280	0.340	1.000	5.28	1892	18917	1.009	0
3	7.150	0.360	1.897	6.15	2187	21873	1.463	0

EXPERIMENT 65

HPLC determination of ciprofloxacin tablet

Ciprofloxacin, a broad-spectrum antiinfective agent of the fluoroquinolone class, is used to treat gram-negative infections, sexually transmitted diseases, mycobacterial infections, corneal ulcers, and bacterial conjunctivitis. For the treatment of bacterial infection of respiratory tract, UTI, uncomplicated cystitis in females, GI, chronic bacterial prostatitis, CNS, immunocompromised patients, skin, bone and joint infections, uncomplicated cervical and urethral gonorrhea.

Ciprofloxacin

Experimental overview

The objective of this experiment is to determine the % of ciprofloxacin base in ciprofloxacin HCl tablet.

The instrument used in this experiment is a Simazdu LC system, consisting of LC-10ATVP pump and SPD-10AVP detector system.

Procedure

HPLC conditions:

Column: C_{18} 250 × 4.6 mm (5 mm).

Mobile phase: 87 volume of 0.025 M phosphoric acid and 13 volume of acetonitrile, pH 3.0 ± 0.1 adjusted with triethylamine.

Flow rate: 2.0 ml/min

Injection volume: 20 µl

Wavelength: 278 nm

(A) **Preparation of solutions:**

    (1) *Standard solution:* Completely dissolve approximately 120 mg of ciprofloxacin HCl in 100ml of mobile phase. Dilute 10 ml of this solution to 100 ml with mobile phase.

    (2) *Test sample:* Weigh and powder 20 tablets. Dissolve about 125 mg of powder with 50 ml of mobile phase, filter and dilute to 100 ml with mobile phase in volumetric flask. Dilute 10 ml of this solution to 100 ml with mobile phase.

(B) **Analysis:**

    (1) Inject the 20 microlitre of standard solution in the HPLC system and run the system following instructor's directions.

    (2) Print a chromatogram and integration information for each sample.

    (3) Similarly, do the same with test sample.

Note: Sample chromatograms of standard and test are enclosed here for reference.

Observation and calculation

Mass of ciprofloxacin HCl (standard): 121.8 mg

Average weight of tablet: 980.3 mg

Weight of powder dissolved in mobile phase: 126.9 mg

Concentration of ciprofloxacin HCl in stock solution: 1.218 mg/ml

Concentration of ciprofloxacin HCl in the standard solutions: 0.012 mg/ml

Molecular weight of ciprofloxacin HCl = 385.8

Molecular weight of ciprofloxacin base = 331.40

% purity of ciprofloxacin HCl = 94%

Ciprofloxacin HCl retention time: 18.01

Ciprofloxacin HCl peak area (in standard): 23560.1197

Ciprofloxacin HCl peak area (in test): 22859.5259

Dilution factor of standard and sample is same.

Calculation based on peak area analysis:

Content of ciprofloxacin base equivalent to ciprofloxacin HCl tablet:

$$= \frac{22859.5 \times 121.8 \times 331.40}{23560.1 \times 126.9 \times 385.8} \times \frac{94}{100} \times 980.3 = 737 \text{ mg (claim 750 mg)}$$

Result

The average weight tablet contains 737 mg of ciprofloxacin base.

Judge yourself

1. What is the general mechanism of high performance liqiud chromatography?
2. What is the use of HPLC? What is the importance in the pharma field?
3. How does HPLC differ from normal column chromatography, and what are its advantages?

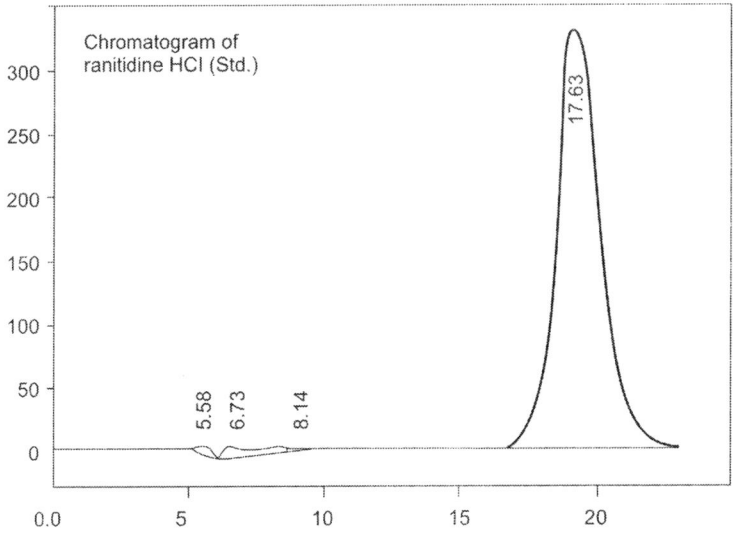

Result

Calculation method Uncal

Peak No.	Reten. time	Area [mV.s]	Height [mV]	W05 [min.]	Area [%]	Height [%]
1	5.580	262.7199	4.0360	1.2500	1.0672	1.1972
2	6.730	480.5540	7.8790	1.2800	1.9520	2.3372
3	8.140	315.3262	4.1308	2.3200	1.2808	1.2253
4	17.630	23560.1197	321.0714	1.1200	95.7000	95.2403
	Total	24618.7098	337.1172			

Column performance test report

Peak No.	Reten. time	W05 [min.]	Asymmetry [–]	Capacity [–]	Efficiency [th. pl.]	Eff./1 [t.p./m]	Resolution [–]	Rct. index [–]
1	5.580	1.250	0.985	4.58	110	1105	–	0
2	6.730	1.280	2.381	5.73	153	1533	0.535	0
3	8.140	2.320	4.146	7.14	68	683	0.461	0
4	17.630	1.120	1.393	16.63	1374	13739	3.248	0

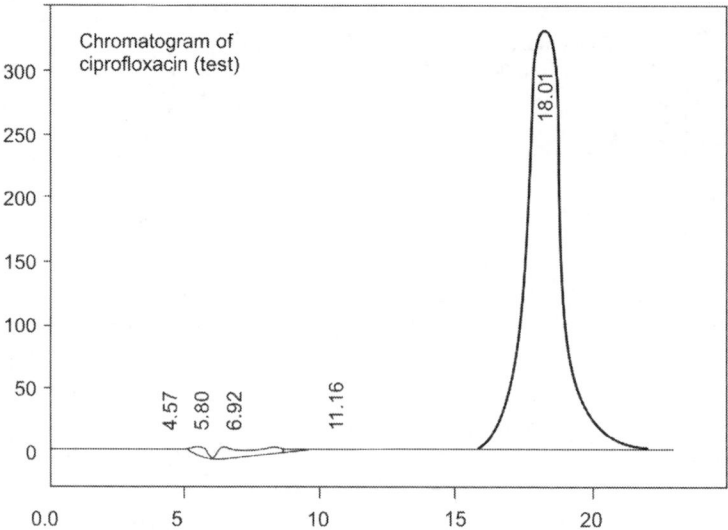

Result

Calculation method Uncal

Peak No.	Reten. time	Area [mV.s]	Height [mV]	W05 [min.]	Area [%]	Height [%]
1	4.670	12.4011	0.7632	0.3100	0.0504	0.2461
2	5.800	344.6801	5.2216	1.3800	1.4004	1.6835
3	6.920	580.0357	10.3496	1.0800	2.3567	3.3368
4	11.160	815.5729	0.6160	1.1100	3.3137	0.1986
5	18.010	22859.5259	293.2181	1.1800	92.8788	94.5350
	Total	24612.2157	310.1685			

Column performance test report

Peak No.	Reten. time	W05 [min.]	Asymmetry [–]	Capacity [–]	Efficiency [th. pl.]	Eff./1 [t.p./m]	Resolution [–]	Ret. index [–]
1	4.670	0.310	1.167	3.67	1258	12584	–	0
2	5.800	1.380	0.785	4.80	98	979	0.787	0
3	6.920	1.080	1.951	5.92	228	2276	0.536	0
4	11.160	1.110	0.070	10.16	561	5605	2.280	0
5	18.010	1.180	1.323	17.01	1292	12917	3.522	0

EXPERIMENT 66

HPLC determination of cetrizine dihydrochloride tablet

Cetirizine dihydrochloride is an orally active and selective H_1-receptor antagonist. The chemical name is (±)–[2–[4–[(4–chlorophenyl)phenylmethyl]–1–piperazinyl]ethoxy]acetic acid, dihydrochloride. Cetirizine hydrochloride is a racemic compound with an empirical formula of $C_{21}H_{25}C_1N_2O_3 \cdot 2HCl$. The molecular weight is 461.82 and the chemical structure is shown below:

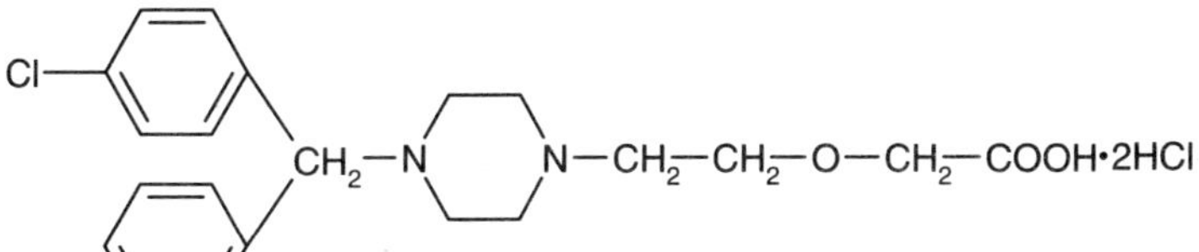

Cetrizine Dihydrochloride

Cetirizine hydrochloride is a white, crystalline powder and is water soluble. The tablets are formulated as white, film-coated, rounded-off rectangular shaped tablets for oral administration and are available in 5 and 10 mg strengths. Inactive ingredients are: lactose monohydrate; microcrystalline cellulose; colloidal silicon dioxide; croscarmellose sodium; magnesium stearate; titanium dioxide; hypromellose; and polyethylene glycol.

Experimental overview

The objective of this experiment is to determine the % of ciprofloxacin base in ciprofloxacin HCl tablet.

The instrument used in this experiment is a Simazdu LC system, consisting of LC-10 ATVP pump and SPD-10AVP detector system.

Procedure

HPLC conditions:

Column: C_{18} 250 × 4.6 mm (5 mm).

Mobile phase: 80 volume of acetonitrile, 19.6 volume of water and 0.4 volume of dilute sulfuric acid.

Flow rate: 0.6 ml/min.

Injection volume: 20 µl.

Wavelength: 230 nm.

(A) **Preparation of solutions:**

(1) *Standard solution*: Completely dissolve approximately 50 mg of cetrizine 2 HCl in 50 ml of water. Dilute 1.0 ml of this solution to 100ml with mobile phase.

(2) *Test sample:* Weigh and powder 20 tablets. Dissolve the powder equivalent to 50 mg of cetrizine 2 HCl in 25 ml of water, filter and dilute to 50 ml with mobile phase in volumetric flask. Dilute 1.0 ml of this solution to 100 ml with mobile phase.

(B) **Analysis:**

(1) Inject the 20 microlitre of standard solution in the HPLC system and run the system following instructor's directions.

(2) Print a chromatogram and integration information for each sample.

(3) Similarly, do the same with test sample.

Note: Sample chromatograms of standard and test are enclosed here for reference.

Observation and calculation

Mass of cetrizine 2HCl (standard): 51.21 mg

Average weight of tablet: 131.0 mg

Weight of powder dissolved in mobile phase: 640.8 mg

Concentration of cetrizine2HCl in stock solution: 1.2 mg/ml

Concentration of cetrizine 2HCl in the standard solutions: 0.012 mg/ml

% purity of cetrizine 2HCl = 99%

Cetrizine 2HCl retention time: 3.91

Cetrizine2HCl peak area (in standard): 7228.2201

Cetrizine2HCl peak area (in test): 6775.8454

Dilution factor of standard and sample is same.

Calculation based on peak area analysis:

$$= \frac{6775 \times 51.21}{7228 \times 640.8} \times \frac{99}{100} \times 131 = 9.71 \, \text{mg (claim 10 mg)}$$

Result

The average weight tablet contains 737 mg of cetrizine 2HCl.

Judge yourself

1. How to choose the flow cell volume for a UV detector?
2. What are important specifications for a column?
3. What are the differences between reverse phase HPLC and normal phase HPLC?
4. Why acetonitrile and methanol are most commonly used solvents for reverse phase HPLC?

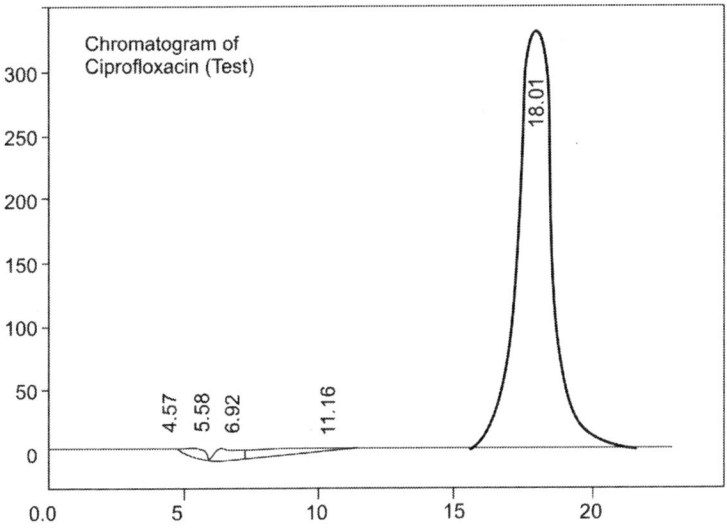

Chromatogram of Ciprofloxacin (Test)

Result

Calculation method Uncal

Peak No.	Reten. time	Area [mV.s]	Height [mV]	W05 [min.]	Area [%]	Height [%]
1	3.450	26.6578	3.2073	0.1000	0.3512	0.7039
2	3.830	7228.2201	440.7819	0.2700	95.2194	96.7382
3	4.630	127.5419	6.7237	0.3900	1.6801	1.4756
4	5.070	197.4442	4.6341	0.5500	2.6010	1.0171
5	9.430	11.2543	0.2972	0.6300	0.1483	0.0652
	Total	7591.1183	455.6442			

Column performance test report

Peak No.	Reten. time	W05 [min.]	Asymmetry [-]	Capacity [-]	Efficiency [th. pl.]	Eff./1 [t.p./m]	Resolution [-]	Ret. index [-]
1	3.450	0.100	0.296	2.45	6600	65999	–	0
2	3.830	0.270	2.154	2.83	1116	11158	1.209	0
3	4.630	0.390	3.333	3.63	78	7815	1.427	0
4	5.070	0.550	10.643	4.07	471	4712	0.551	0
5	9.430	0.630	3.714	8.43	1242	12423	4.350	0

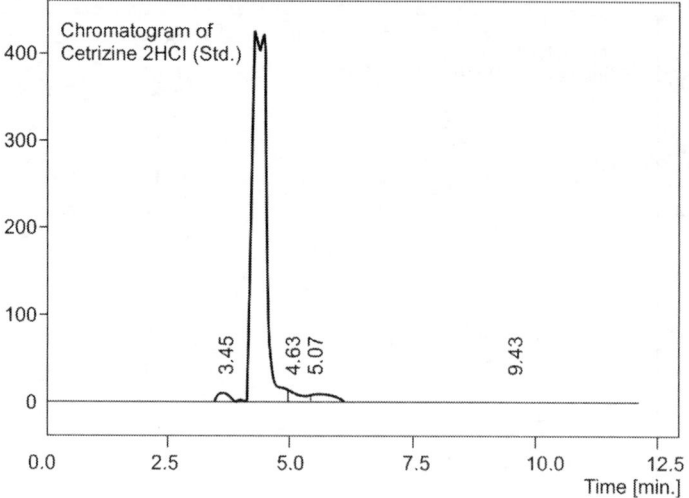

Result

Calculation method Uncal

Peak No.	Reten. time	Area [mV.s]	Height [mV]	W05 [min.]	Area [%]	Height [%]
1	3.430	54.0521	5.9726	0.1200	0.7726	1.4645
2	3.910	6775.8454	390.7078	0.2900	96.8521	95.8034
3	5.060	74.8980	6.5331	0.2100	1.0706	1.6020
4	5.280	91.2783	4.6088	0.3500	1.3047	1.1301
	Total	6996.0738	407.8223			

Column performance test report

Peak No.	Reten. time	W05 [min.]	Asymmetry [–]	Capacity [–]	Efficiency [th. pl.]	Eff./1 [t.p./m]	Resolution [–]	Ret. index [–]
1	3.430	0.120	0.333	2.43	4530	45303	–	0
2	3.910	0.290	0.846	2.91	1008	10080	–	0
3	5.060	0.210	0.765	4.06	3219	32193	2.708	0
4	5.280	0.350	4.556	4.28	1262	12619	0.463	0

EXPERIMENT 67

HPLC determination of omeprazole capsules

Omeprazole is a proton pump inhibitor used in the treatment of dyspepsia, peptic ulcer disease (PUD), gastroesophageal reflux disease and Zollinger-Ellison syndrome. It was first marketed in the US in 1989 by Astra Zeneca as the magnesium salt **omeprazole magnesium** under the brand names **Losec** and **Prilosec**, and is now also available from generic manufacturers under various brand names. Omeprazole is one of the most widely prescribed drugs internationally and is available over the counter in some countries.

Omeprazole

Omeprazole is a white to off-white crystalline powder that melts with decomposition at about 155°C. It is a weak base, freely soluble in ethanol and methanol, and slightly soluble in acetone and isopropanol and very slightly soluble in water. The stability of omeprazole is a function of pH; it is rapidly degraded in acid media, but has acceptable stability under alkaline conditions.Omeprazole is available as tablets and capsules (containing omeprazole or omeprazole magnesium) in strengths of 10 mg, 20 mg, and in some markets 40 mg.

Experimental overview

The objective of this experiment is to determine the % of ciprofloxacin base in ciprofloxacin HCl tablet.

The instrument used in this experiment is a Simazdu LC system, consisting of LC-10ATVP pump and SPD-10AVP detector system.

Procedure

HPLC conditions:

Column: C_{18} 250 × 4.6 mm (5 mm).

Mobile phase: 65 volume of 0.05 M Disodium hydrogen orthophosphate and 35 volume of acetonitrile, pH djusted to 6.5 with orthophosphoric acid.

Flow rate: 0.8 ml/min.

Injection volume: 20 µl.

Wavelength: 302 nm.

(A) **Preparation of solutions:**

(1) *Standard solution*: Completely dissolve approximately 266 mg of omeprazole in 0.1 M NaOH solution. Dilute 5.0 ml of this solution to 25.0 ml with mobile phase.

(2) *Test sample*: Weigh and powder 20 capsules. Dissolve the approximately 266 mg powder in 40ml of 0.1 M NaOH solution, filter and dilute to 50ml in volumetric flask. Dilute 5.0 ml of this solution to 25.0 ml with mobile phase.

(B) **Analysis:**

(1) Inject the 20 microlitre of standard solution in the HPLC system and run the system following instructor's directions.

(2) Print a chromatogram and integration information for each sample.

(3) Similarly, do the same with test sample.

Note: Sample chromatograms of standard and test are enclosed here for reference.

Observation and calculation

Mass of omeprazole (standard): 266.4 mg

Average weight of tablet: 300.0 mg

Weight of powder dissolved in mobile phase: 268.5 mg

Concentration of omeprazole in stock solution: 5.32 mg/ml

Concentration of omeprazole in the standard solutions: 0.21 mg/ml

% purity of omeprazole = 7.5%

Note: Omeprazole comes as pellet, containing 7.5% of omeprazole. These are packed into capsule shell along with excepients.

Omeprazole retention time: 3.91

Omeprazole peak area (in standard): 9171.3595

Omeprazole peak area (in test): 9080.0617

Dilution factor of standard and sample is same.

Calculation based on peak area analysis:

$$= \frac{9080.06 \times 266.4}{9171.35 \times 268.5} \times \frac{7.5}{100} \times 300 = 19.84 \text{ mg (claim 20 mg)}$$

Result

The average weight tablet contains 19.84 mg of omeprazole.

Judge yourself

1. What are the basic components for a HPLC system?
2. There are so many brands of HPLC available in the market, how do you judge which one is the best for me?
3. How many types of detectors are available for HPLC?

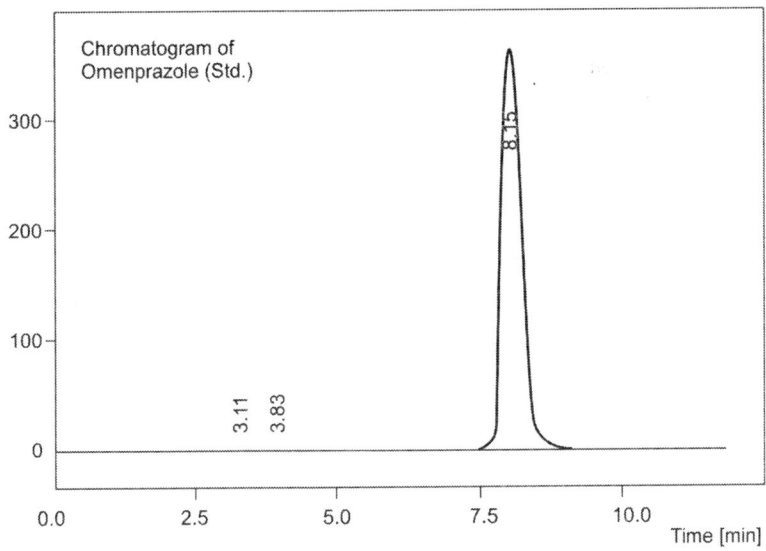

Chromatogram of Omenprazole (Std.)

Result

Calculation method Uncal

Peak No.	Reten. time	Area [mV.s]	Height [mV]	W05 [min.]	Area [%]	Height [%]
1	3.110	20.5922	0.8131	0.4100	0.2215	0.2191
2	3.830	105.3259	3.9573	0.2600	1.1329	1.0775
3	8.150	9171.3595	366.2896	0.3500	98.6456	98.7144
	Total	9297.2776	371.0600			

Column performance test report

Peak No.	Reten. time	W05 [min.]	Asymmetry [–]	Capacity [–]	Efficiency [th. pl.]	Eff./1 [t.p./m]	Resolution [–]	Ret. index [–]
1	3.110	0.410	0.860	2.11	319	3190	–	0
2	3.830	0.260	1.560	2.83	1203	12032	1.265	0
5	8.150	0.350	0.929	7.15	3007	30066	8.338	0

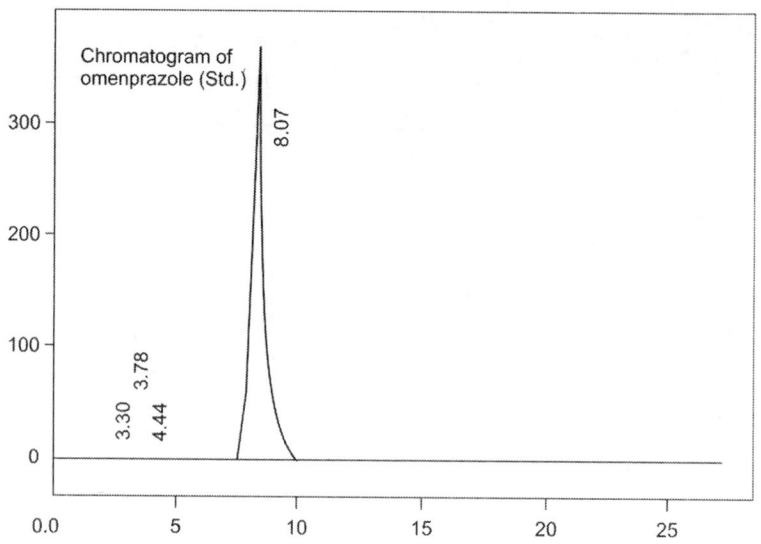

Result

Calculation method Uncal

Peak No.	Reten. time	Area [mV.s]	Height [mV]	W05 [min.]	Area [%]	Height [%]
1	3.330	14.8525	0.6987	0.3300	0.1620	0.1881
2	3.780	51.0890	3.2286	0.2300	0.5571	0.8692
3	4.440	24.0035	0.3034	0.9700	0.2618	0.0817
4	8.070	9080.0617	367.2198	0.3400	99.0191	98.8610
	Total	9170.0067	371.4505			

Column performance test report

Peak No.	Reten. time	W05 [min.]	Asymmetry [–]	Capacity [–]	Efficiency [th. pl.]	Eff./1 [t.p./m]	Resolution [–]	Ret. index [–]
1	3.330	0.330	0.788	2.30	555	5545	–	0
2	3.780	0.230	1.500	2.78	1498	14977	1.009	0
3	4.440	0.970	10.714	3.44	116	1162	0.648	0
4	8.070	0.340	0.951	7.07	3124	31239	3.263	0

Differential Scanning Colorimetry

Introduction

Differential scanning calorimetry (DSC) is one of the analytical techniques belonging to a group called thermal analysis (TA). They involve measuring changes of various physical quantities with changing temperature, e.g.

Technique	Measured quantity
DTA—Differential Thermal Analysis	Temperature difference (between sample and reference)
DSC—Differential Scanning Calorimetry	Heat difference (between sample and reference)
TG—Thermogravimetry	Mass
TMA—Thermomechanical Analysis	Dimensions

The **applications** of DSC include:

- Phase transition definition including melting point, glass transition, Curie point
- Determination of crystallinity
- Kinetic studies
- Material fingerprinting

Theory

The idea of a DSC experiment is to heat up or cool down a sample and a reference according to a set temperature programme. The sample and reference are maintained at the same temperature during the whole experiment. When a thermal event occurs in the sample, certain, additional amount of energy has to be supplied to or withdrawn from the sample to maintain zero temperature difference between the sample and the reference. Therefore, the reference should not undergo any physical or chemical changes at the temperature range of the experiment. The sample and reference are placed in identical environments—metal pans on individual bases, each of which contains a platinum resistance thermometer (or a thermocouple) and a heater (Fig. 17.1). An empty pan is very often used as a reference. The temperatures of the two thermometers are compared and the electric power supplied to each heater adjusted so that the temperatures of the sample and the reference remain equal, i.e. any temperature difference which would result from a thermal event in the sample is compensated for. If an exothermic change occurs in the sample, more heat has to be supplied to the reference (which is equivalent to withdrawing energy from the sample). During an endothermic process, additional amount of energy has to be supplied to the sample heater. The difference in the

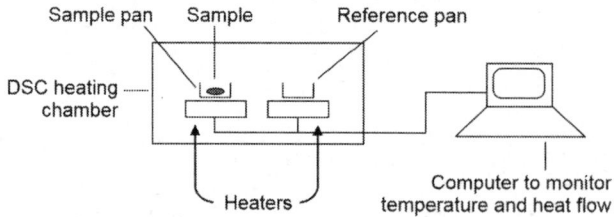

Fig. 17.1: DSC experimental setup.

heat supplied to the sample and the reference is recorded as a function of temperature. This signal is proportional to the sample specific heat, which determines the amount of heat that is necessary to change the sample temperature by a given amount.

Any transition that is accompanied by a change in specific heat produces a variation in the power signal. Exothermic and endothermic processes give peaks with areas proportional to the total enthalpy change of the events (Fig. 17.2).

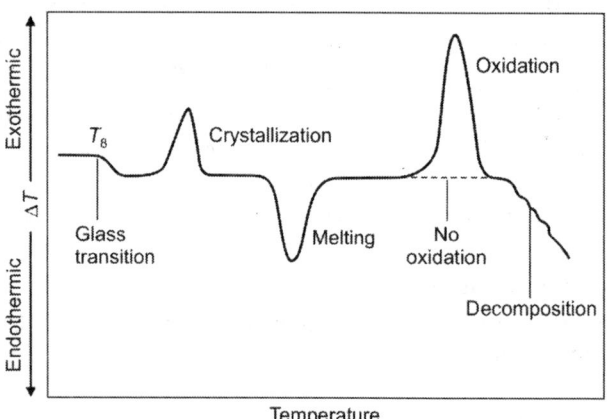

Fig. 17.2: A typical DSC curve.

Summing up, the measuring principle in DSC is to compare the rate of heat flow to a sample and to a reference. Both the sample and the reference are heated or cooled at the same rate and their temperatures are maintained at the same level. Changes in the sample that are associated with absorption or evolution of heat cause variations in the differential heat flow which are then recorded as peaks, The area of an individual peak is directly proportional to the enthalpy change of the sample and the direction of the peak indicates whether the thermal event is exo- or endothermic.

Purity determination by DSC

Historically, it has been observed that freezing points are depressed when impurities are present in a material, and later, pre-melting on re-heating an impure material was noted. With the introduction of the DSC, a method of quantifying the levels of impurity by differential scanning calorimetry was derived. The purity calculation in differential scanning calorimetry is applied to materials that are pure crystalline materials (i.e. discrete compounds) rather than polymeric materials or mixtures. Indeed, the purity of the material being analyzed should not be lower than 95 mole % (mol%). Below this level, the assumptions made in the calculation are not valid; preferably, the purity of the material under examination should be greater than 97 mol% so that errors are minimized. The purity calculation works by analyzing the rate of melting of the sample, and from this, determining the depression of the melting point, which is caused by the presence of the impurity.

The melting transitions of a pure 100% crystalline material should be infinitely sharp, but impurities or defects in the crystal structure will broaden the melting range (Fig. 17.3) and lower the final melting point to a temperature lower than T_0. The effect of impurities is determined by DSC method based on van't Hoff equation (17. 1).

$$\Delta T = \frac{RT_0^2 X_2}{\Delta H} \qquad \dots(17.1)$$

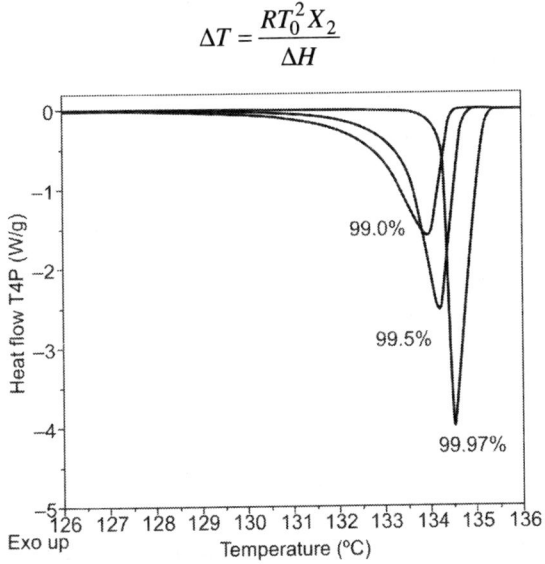

Fig. 17.3: DSC melting curves of phenacetin at three purity levels.

or

$$X_2 = \frac{\Delta T \times \Delta H}{RT_0^2}$$

where,

ΔH = Heat of fusion (J mg^{-1}, calculated from peak area)

R = Gas constant

ΔT = Change in sample temperature

X_2 = Mole fraction of impurities

T_0 = Theoretical melting point of pure compound

EXPERIMENT 68

To determine the purity of paracetamol/acetaminophen in standard preparation by using differential scanning calorimeter (DSC)

Requirements

- Phase transition definition including melting point, glass transition, Curie point
- DSC instrument
- Pure paracetamol (API)
- Marketed formulation of paracetamol
- Degassing equipment/N_2 gas assembly
- Methanol AR grade

Procedure

Standard preparation

- Weigh an empty sample pan and cover.
- Add the sample accurately about 5mg of pure paracetamol into an aluminium pan and crimped a lid and reweigh. Use an analytical balance or micro-balance with an accuracy of at least ±0.02 mg.
- Crimp the pan, If any aluminum is lost during crimping, reweigh the crimped sample-pan-lid. An empty pan and lid are always kept in the reference holder.
- Obtain the Thermogram over the temperature range 25–60°C, with a 20°C min^{-1} scan rate.
- Choose a scan RANGE setting so that the baseline before and after the starting transient are both between 0 and 10 mV.
- Repeat the DSC scan(s) using the same parameters as in 1. (Depending on circumstances, it may be useful to do repeat scans with the same sample to establish reversibility and reproducibility.)
- After final cooling, remove the sample and examine for weight loss.
- Process data using instrumental software.

Sample preparation

- Branded tablet formulation of paracetamol is crushed and dissolved in methanol and sonicated for 30 minutes.
- Then filtered by Whatman filter paper (0.45 µ) and filtrate is dried to get about 5 mg of residue.
- This residue will be analysed for DSC like standard paracetamol as explained above.

Observation from DSC thermogram

A thermogram records the heat flow into or out of the sample versus time or temperature. In the thermogram above heat flow in milliwatts (mW or mJ/s)) is plotted versus temperature. A negative peak corresponds to heat absorption or an endothermic process, and a positive peak corresponds to heat evolution or an exothermic process.

This thermogram shows the melting of paracetamol, an endothermic process. The enthalpy of the process is given by the area under the peak. From the thermogram, the enthalpy of fusion of paracetamol, is 165.58 J g^{-1}, and the melting point (the onset temperature) is 167.89°C.

The purity of sample paracetamol is calculataed from the sample thermogram by use of modified form of van't Hoff equation, i.e.

$$\Delta T = \frac{RT_0^2 X_2}{\Delta H} \qquad \qquad ...(17.1)$$

or

$$X_2 = \frac{\Delta T \times \Delta H}{RT_0^2}$$

where,

ΔH = Heat of fusion (J mg^{-1}, calculated from peak area)

R = Gas constant

ΔT = Change in sample temperature

X_2 = Mole fraction of impurities

T_0 = Theoretical melting point of pure compound

Obsevation and calculation

For standard paracetamol

Peak = 171.403°C

ΔH = 660.509J/g

Area = 660.509 mJ

Temp = 167.638°C

For sample paracetamol

Peak = 175.370°C

ΔH = 2195.002 J/g

Area = 2195.002 mJ

ΔT = 175.370 -171.403

Temp = 167.638°C

$$X_2 = \frac{\Delta T \times \Delta H}{RT_0^2}$$

$$X_2 = \frac{(175.370 - 171.403) \times (2195 - 660)}{8.314 \times 167.638^2}$$

$$= \frac{6089}{8.314 \times 29378}$$

$$= \frac{6089}{244256}$$

$$= 0.0249$$

% purity = 100 − 0.0249= 99.975%

Result

The % purity of standard paracetamol formulation is found to be 99.975% by using differential scanning calorimeter (DSC).

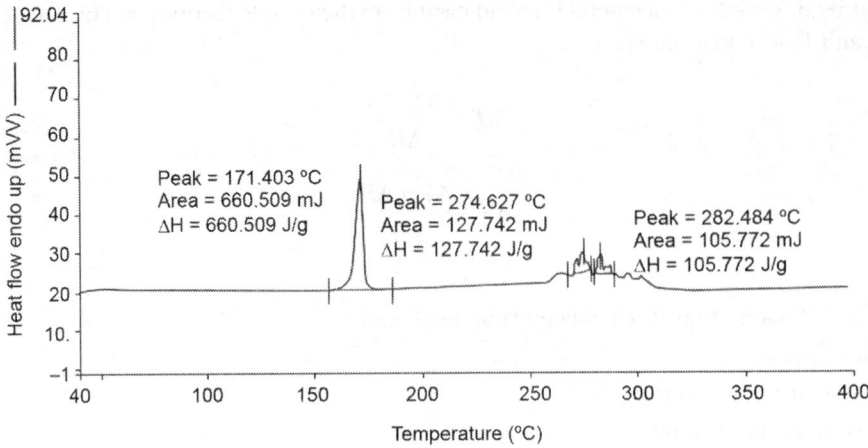

Fig. 17.4: Thermogram of paracetamol (reference).

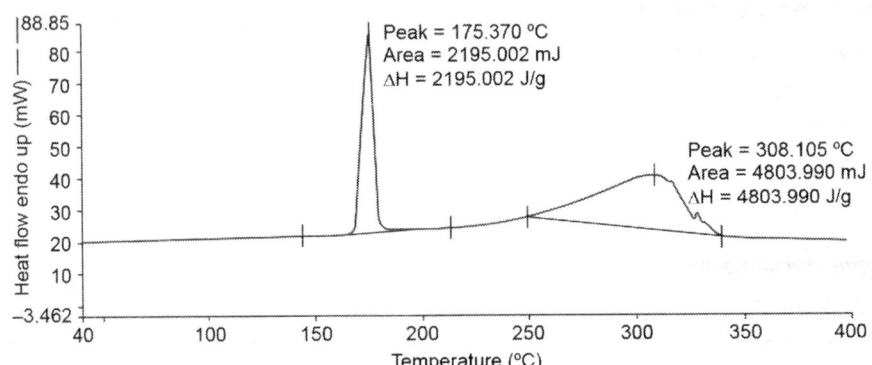

Fig. 17.5: Thermogram of paracetamol (sample).

Judge yourself

1. What is the unit of enthalpy?
2. What is the difference between thermogram and thermograph?
3. How much amount is used for DSC analysis?
4. DCS calculation is based on which equation?
5. What conclusions we are going to get from DSC thermogram?

High Performance
Thin Layer Chromatography

High performance thin layer chromatography (HPTLC) is a sophisticated instrumental technique based on the full capabilities of thin layer chromatography. The basic principle of TLC and HPTLC is same (adsorption and partition of solute between stationary phase and mobile phase). The HPTLC can be used as qualitative and quantitative tool for sample analysis/identification however the TLC is only qualitative method for sample identification.

In HPTLC, sample is injected (0.1 to 10 microliter) on to the silica plate using an auto-injector inbuilt with a syringe with the help of inert gas (N_2 gas). At a time 10 to 15 samples can be spotted on the silica plate keeping a minimum distance between each sample.

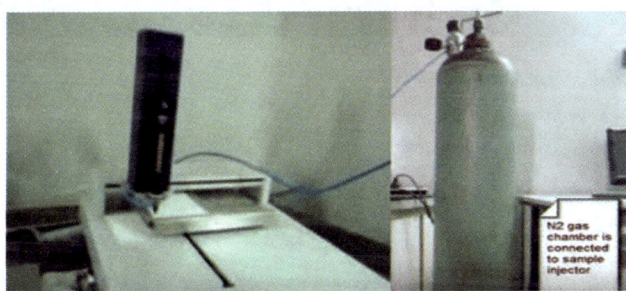

Once the sample is injected onto the silica plate, it is kept inside the saturated chamber for chromatogram to express with different pattern of sample(s).

On completion of chromatogram expression (TLC plate), it is kept inside the visualizer (densitometer) to review it at different wavelength (254 nm or 366 nm).

Compounds due to absence of chromophores, are either UV inactive or show very week UV band. In such cases, the TLC plate is sprayed with some derivatising reagent that forms a complex with the compound present on to the plate and hence become UV active. The TLC plate then can be visulize inside the densitometer with prominent band(s).

With the help of inbuilt computer software, these TLC plates can be converted into a virtual peak that would be having area count corresponding to its concentration. In general, low intense spot would has low area count and high intense spot has high area count. It is to be noted that, distance travel by a particular compound would be similar however its area count would be variable depending on its concentration. The software convert the TLC plate into a peak chromatogram as well as it also represents it in three dimensional view.

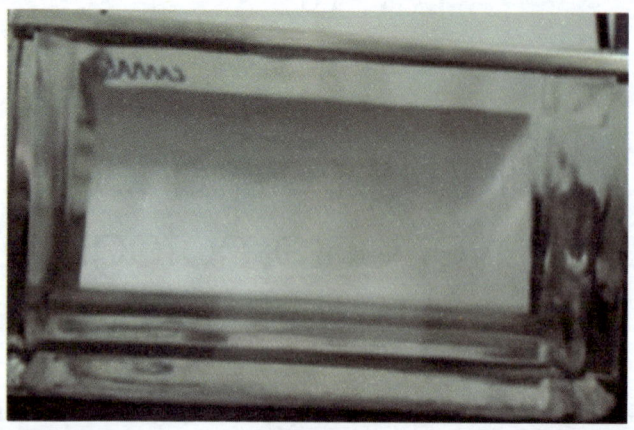

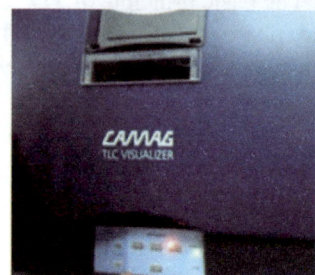 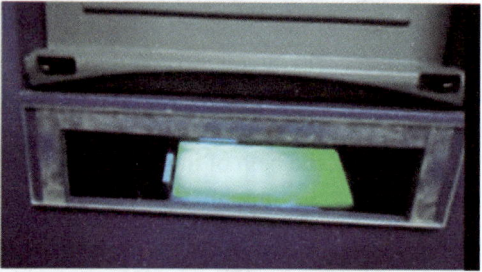

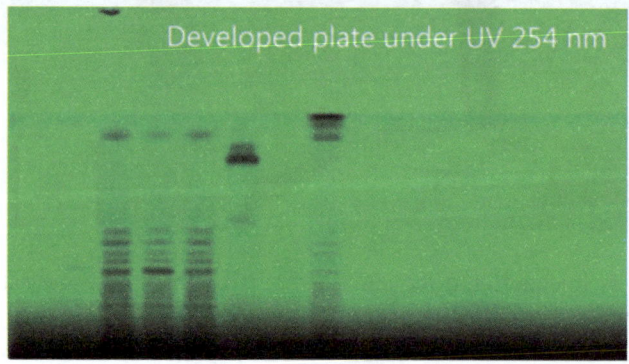

Developed plate under UV 254 nm

Example of typical chromatogram at 254 nm

A typical example has been shown below where TLC plate has been subjected to 254 nm, 366 nm and in normal day light after derivatization:

Just like any other quantitative technique, HPTLC technique also needs to be developed and validated before going for sample analysis. There are various parameters (Selectivity, sensitivity, person, accuracy, ruggedness, recovery) that are required to validate during method development and validation.

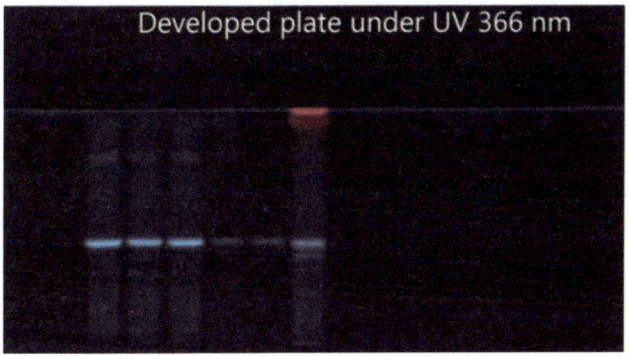

Example of typical chromatogram at 366 nm

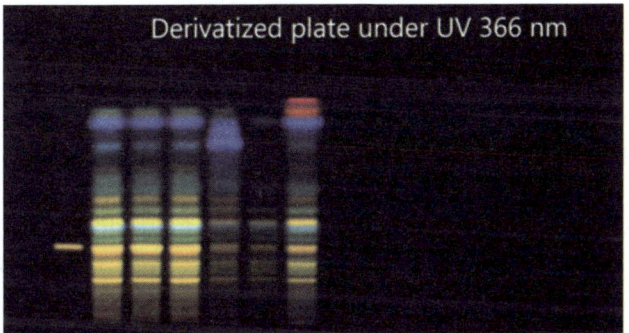

Example of typical chromatogram at 366 nm after derivatization

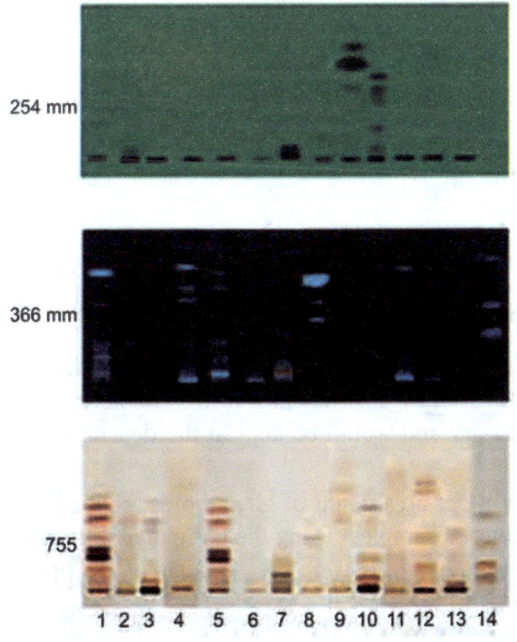

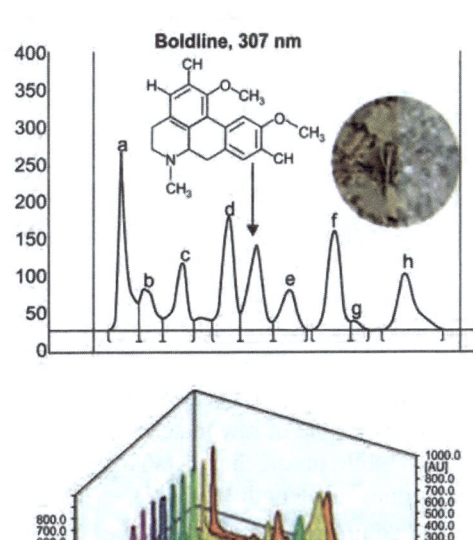

EXPERIMENT 69

To analyse the diphenhydramine hydrochloride concentration in a pharmaceutical raw materials (PRM)

Diphenhydramine is an antihistamine used to relieve symptoms of allergy, hay fever, and the common cold. These symptoms include rash, itching, watery eyes, itchy eyes/nose/throat, cough, runny nose, and sneezing. It is also used to prevent and treat nausea, vomiting and dizziness caused by motion sickness.

Diphenhydramine hydrochloride

Experimental procedure

For qualitative analysis, we need to prepare a standard solution of diphenhydramine hydrochloride ($C_{17}H_{21}NO.HCl$, mol. wt. 291.82) by weighing it 1 mg/1 ml in methanol followed by making its calibration curve (CC) concentrations (1, 2, 15, 30, 60, 80, 100 and 120 ng/ml).

1 mg/ml = 1000 µg/ml or 1,000,000 ng/ml

Stock conc. (ng/ml)	Volume taken (ml)	Volume upto (ml)	Final conc. (ng/ml)
1,000,000	1.00	100	10000
10,000	1.20	100	120
10,000	1.00	100	100
10,000	0.80	100	80
10,000	0.60	100	60
10,000	0.30	100	30
10,000	0.15	100	15
15	1.00	10	2
2	5	10	1

Now these samples (calibration curve need to be spiked on to the TLC plate along with one unknown sample of raw material using auto injector of HPTLC instrument followed by keeping it in the mobile phase chamber. This TLC plate need to dry and would be kept in the densitometer under one wavelength (254 nm).

On completion of assessment of TLC plate we will get area count of all samples (calibration curve standards and unknown pharmaceutical raw material samples) using the computer software.

Since the linear regression has been used for the method, hence we can back calculate the PRM sample concentration using linear equation:

$$Y = mX + C$$

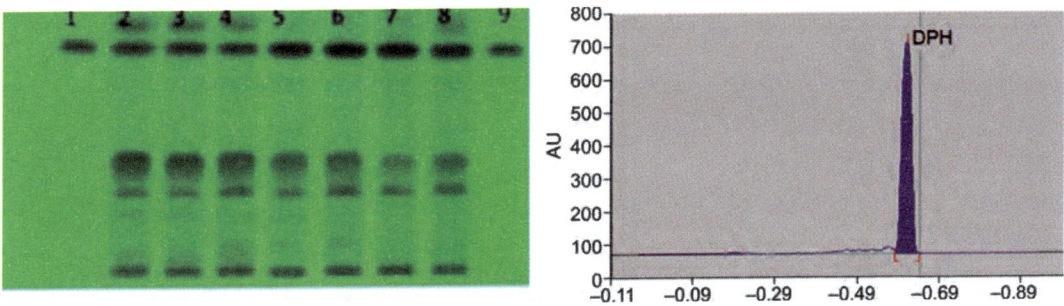

TLC chromatogram of STDs and unknown TLC chromatogram of unknown at 254nm

where Y = Area count of sample

m = Slope

X = Concentration generated by software

C = Intercept

S. No.	Sample	Area counts (at 254 nm)	Linear regression equation
1.	CC (1 ng/ml)	3009	
2.	CC (2 ng/ml)	6424	$y = 166x + (-304)$
3.	CC (15 ng/ml)	162590	$(r = 0.9995)$
4.	CC (30 ng/ml)	342510	
5.	CC (60 ng/ml)	673144	
6.	CC (80 ng/ml)	889715	
7.	CC (100 ng/ml)	1076690	
8.	CC (120 ng/ml)	1279692	
			Calculation for concentration $[y - (-304)]/166 = x$
9.	Diphenhydramine hydrochloride	3051	$[3051 - (-304)]/166 = 20.21$ ng/ml

Generated by software

Result

The unknown concentration of diphenhydramine hydrochloride in pharmaceutical raw material is 20.21 ng/ml.

Judge yourself

1. What is the concept of HPTLC?
2. What are quantitative applications of HPTLC?
3. Mention the derivatizing agents used in HPTLC.
4. What UV wavelength is used in HPTLC analysis?

Appendices

APPENDIX I

VOLUMETRIC SOLUTIONS

Primary standard: A primary standard is a highly pure (at least 99.99%) compound that serves as reference material in all volumetric methods For example, oxalic acid dihydrate is a primary standard, used to determine the concentration of a standard solution of NaOH (with approximate concentration).

Requirements for primary standard:
- Usually solid to make it easier to weigh.
- Easy to obtain, purify and store, and easy to dry.
- Inert in the atmosphere.
- High formula weight so that it can be weighed with high precision.

Primary standard in common use:

$$K_2Cr_2O_7;\ Na_2C_2O_4;\ H_2C_2O_4.2H_2O;\ Na_2B_4O_7.10H_2O;\ CaCO_3;\ NaCl;\ Na_2CO_3$$

Normal solutions: Normal solutions contain 1 g equivalent weight of the active substance in 1 litre of solution; that is, an amount equivalent to 1.0079 g of hydrogen or 7.9997 g of oxygen. Normal solutions and solutions bearing a specific relationship to normal solutions, and used in volumetric determinations, are designated as follows: Normal, 1 N; double-normal, 2 N; half-normal, 0.5 N; tenth-normal, 0.1 N; fiftieth-normal, 0.02 N; hundredth-normal, 0.01 N; thousandth-normal, 0.001 N.

Molar solutions: Molar solutions contain, in 1 litre, 1 g molecule of the reagent. Thus, each litre of a molar solution of sulfuric acid contains 98.07 g of H_2SO_4 and each litre of a molar solution of potassium ferricyanide contains 329.25 g of $K_3Fe(CN)_6$. Solutions containing, in 1 litre, one-tenth of a gram-molecule of the reagent are designated "tenth-molar", 0.1 M; and other molarities are similarly indicated.

Empirical solutions: It is frequently difficult to prepare standard solutions of a desired theoretical normality, and this is not essential. A solution of approximately the desired normality is prepared and standardized by titration against a primary standard solution. The normality factor so obtained is used in all calculations where such empirical solutions are employed. If desired, an empirically prepared solution may be adjusted downward to a given normality provided it is strong enough to permit dilution.

All volumetric solutions, whether made by direct solution or by dilution of a stronger solution, must be thoroughly mixed by shaking before standardization. As the strength of a standard solution may change upon standing, the factor should be redetermined frequently.

When solutions of a reagent are used in several normalities, the details of the preparation and standardization are usually given for the normality most frequently required. Stronger or weaker solutions are prepared and standardized in the same general manner as described, using proportionate amounts of the reagent. It is possible in many instances to prepare lower normalities accurately by making an exact dilution of a stronger solution. Volumetric solutions prepared by dilution should be restandardized either as directed for the stronger solution or by comparison with another volumetric solution having a known ratio of the stronger solution.

Dilute solutions that are not stable, as, for instance, potassium permanganate 0.01 N and more dilute sodium thiosulfate, are preferably prepared by exactly diluting the higher normality with thoroughly boiled and cooled water on the same day they are required for use.

Standard solution: The standard solution is a solution for which the concentration (molarity) is accurately known.

Blank determinations: Where it is directed that "any necessary correction" be made by a blank determination, the determination is to be conducted with the use of the same quantities of the same reagents treated in the same manner as the solution or mixture containing the portion of the substance under assay or test, but with the substance itself omitted. Appropriate blank corrections are to be made for all official titrimetric assays.

All official assays that are volumetric in nature indicate the weight of the substance being assayed to which each ml of the primary volumetric solution is equivalent. In general, these equivalents may be derived by simple calculation.

Preparation and methods of standardization of volumetric solutions

The following directions give only one method for standardization, but other methods of standardization, capable of yielding at least the same degree of accuracy, may be used. The values obtained in the standardization of volumetric solutions are valid for all pharmacopeial uses of these solutions, regardless of the instrumental or chemical indicators employed in the individual monographs. Where the apparent normality or molarity of a titrant depends upon the special conditions of its use, the individual monograph sets forth the directions for standardizing the reagent in the specified context .For those salts, that usually are available as certified primary standards, or that are available as highly purified salts of primary standard quality, it is permissible to prepare solutions by accurately weighing a suitable quantity of the salt and dissolving it to produce a specific volume of solution of known concentration. Acetic, hydrochloric, and sulfuric acids may be standardized against a sodium hydroxide solution that has recently been standardized against a certified primary standard.

All volumetric solutions, if practicable, are to be prepared, standardized, and used at the standard temperature of 25°. If a titration is carried out with the volumetric solution at a markedly different temperature, standardize the volumetric solution used as the titrant at that different temperature, or make a suitable temperature correction.

> ### Acetic acid (2 M or 2 N)
> $C_2H_4O_2$ 60.05
> 120.10 g in 1000 ml

Add 116 ml of glacial acetic acid to sufficient water to make 1000 ml after cooling to room temperature.

> ### Ammonium thiocyanate, tenth: Normal (0.1 M or 0.1 N)
> NH_4SCN 76.12
> 7.612 g in 1000 ml

Dissolve about 8 g of ammonium thiocyanate in 1000 ml of water, and standardize the solution as follows.

Measure accurately about 30 ml of 0.1 M/0.1 N silver nitrate into a glass-stoppered flask. Dilute with 50 ml of water, then add 2 ml of nitric acid and 2 ml of ferric ammonium sulfate, and titrate with the ammonium thiocyanate solution to the first appearance of a red-brown color. Calculate the normality.

If desirable, 0.1 M ammonium thiocyanate may be replaced by 0.1 M potassium thiocyanate where the former is directed in various tests and assays.

> ### Bromine (0.1 N or 0.05 M)
> Br 79.90
> 7.990 g in 1000 ml

Dissolve 3 g of potassium bromate and 15 g of potassium bromide in water to make 1000 ml, and standardize the solution as follows.

Measure accurately about 25 ml of the solution into a 500 ml iodine flask, and dilute with 120 ml of water. Add 5 ml of hydrochloric acid, insert the stopper in the flask, and shake it gently. Then add 5 ml of potassium iodide TS, again insert the stopper, shake the mixture, allow it to stand for 5 minutes, and titrate the liberated iodine with 0.1 N sodium thiosulfate, adding 3 ml of starch mucilage indicator as the endpoint is approached. Calculate the normality/molarity. Preserve in dark amber-colored, glass-stoppered bottles.

> ### Ceric ammonium nitrate (0.05 N or 0.05 M)
> $Ce(NO_3)_4.2NH_4NO_3$ 548.22
> 2.741 g in 100 ml

Dissolve 2.75 g of ceric ammonium nitrate in 1 N nitric acid to obtain 100 ml of solution, and filter. Standardize the solution as follows.

Measure accurately 10 ml of freshly standardized 0.1 N or 0.1 M ferrous ammonium sulfate into a flask, and dilute with water to about 100 ml. Add 1 drop of ferroin indicator and titrate with the ceric ammonium nitrate solution to a colorless endpoint. From the volume of 0.1 N or 0.1 M ferrous ammonium sulfate (vs. ?) taken and the volume of ceric ammonium nitrate solution consumed, calculate the normality/molarity.

> **Ceric sulfate (0.1 N or 0.1 M)**
>
> $Ce(SO_4)_2$ 332.24
>
> 33.22 g in 1000 ml

Transfer 59 g of ceric ammonium nitrate to a beaker, add 31 ml of sulfuric acid, mix, and cautiously add water, in 20 ml portions, until solution is complete. Cover the beaker, allow to stand overnight, filter through a fine-porosity, sintered-glass crucible, dilute with water to 1000 ml, and mix. Standardize the solution as follows. [**Note:** Prepare the osmium tetroxide solution used in this procedure in a well-ventilated hood, as poisonous vapors are given off by this compound.] Weigh accurately 200 mg of arsenic trioxide, previously dried at 105° for 1 hour, and transfer to a 500 ml conical flask. Wash down the inner walls of the flask with 25 ml of sodium hydroxide solution (2 in 25), swirl to dissolve the substance, and when solution is complete, add 100 ml of water, and mix. Add 10 ml of dilute sulfuric acid (1 in 3), then add 2 drops each of *ortho*-phenanthroline and a 1 in 400 solution of osmium tetroxide in 0.1 N sulfuric acid/0.05 M sulfuric acid, and slowly titrate with the ceric sulfate solution until the pink color is changed to a very pale blue. Calculate the normality/molarity. Each 4.946 mg of arsenic trioxide is equivalent to 1 ml of 0.1 N ceric sulfate.

Standard dichlorophenol-indophenol solution

To 50 mg of 2,6-dichlorophenol-indophenol sodium that has been stored in a desiccator over soda lime add 50 ml of water containing 42 mg of sodium bicarbonate, shake vigorously, and when the dye is dissolved, add water to make 200 ml. Filter into an amber, glass-stoppered bottle. Standardize the solution as follows.

Accurately weigh 50 mg of ascorbic acid RS, and transfer to a glass-stoppered, 50 ml volumetric flask with the aid of a sufficient volume of metaphosphoric-acetic acids to make 50 ml. Immediately transfer 2 ml of the ascorbic acid solution to a 50 ml conical flask containing 5 ml of the metaphosphoric-acetic acids, and titrate rapidly with the dichlorophenol-indophenol solution until a distinct rose-pink color persists for at least 5 seconds. Perform a blank titration by titrating 7 ml of the metaphosphoric-acetic acids plus a volume of water equal to the volume of the dichlorophenol solution used in titrating the ascorbic acid solution. Express the concentration of the standard solution in terms of its equivalent in mg of ascorbic acid.

> **Edetate disodium (0.05 M)**
>
> $C_{10}H_{14}N_2Na_2O_8 \cdot 2H_2O$ 372.24
>
> 18.61 g in 1000 ml

Dissolve 18.6 g of edetate disodium in water to make 1000 ml, and standardize the solution as follows.

Accurately weigh about 200 mg of calcium carbonate, previously dried at 110° for 2 hours and cooled in a desiccator, transfer to a 400 ml beaker, add 10 ml of water, and swirl to form a slurry. Cover the beaker with a watch glass, and introduce 2 ml of diluted hydrochloric acid from a pipet inserted between the lip of the beaker and the edge of the watch glass. Swirl the contents of the beaker to dissolve the calcium carbonate. Wash down the sides of the beaker, the outer surface of the pipet, and the watch glass with water, and dilute with water to about 100 ml. While stirring the solution, preferably with a magnetic stirrer, add about 30 ml of the edetate disodium solution from a 50 ml buret. Add 15 ml of sodium hydroxide and 300 mg of hydroxy naphthol blue, and continue the titration with the edetate disodium solution to a blue endpoint. Calculate the molarity taken by the formula.

$$W/(100.09\ V)$$

in which W is !he weight, in mg, of $CaCO_3$ in the portion of calcium carbonate taken, and V is the volume, in ml, of edetate disodium solution consumed.

Ferric ammonium sulfate (0.1 M or 0.1 N)

$FeNH_4(SO_4)_2 \cdot 12H_2O$ 482.19

48.22 g in 1000 ml

Dissolve 50 g of ferric ammonium sulfate in a mixture of 300 ml of water and 6 ml of sulfuric acid, dilute with water to 1000 ml, and mix. Standardize the solution as follows.

Measure accurately about 40 ml of the solution into a glass-stoppered flask, add 5 ml of hydrochloric acid, mix, and add a solution of 3 g of potassium iodide in 10 ml of water. Insert the stopper, allow to stand for 10 minutes, then titrate the liberated iodine with 0.1 N or 0.1 M sodium thiosulfate, adding 3 ml of starch mucilage indicator as the endpoint is approached. Correct for a blank run on the same quantities of the same reagents, and calculate the normality/molarity.

Store in tight containers, protected from light.

Ferrous ammonium sulfate (0.1 M or 0.1 N)

$Fe(NH_4)_2(SO_4)_2 \cdot 6H_2O$ 392.14

39.21 g in 1000 ml

Dissolve 40 g of ferrous ammonium sulfate in a previously cooled mixture of 40 ml of sulfuric acid and 200 ml of water, dilute with water to 1000 ml, and mix. On the day of use, standardize the solution as follows.

Measure accurately 25 to 30 ml of the solution into a flask, add 2 drops of *ortho*-phenanthroline indicator, and titrate with 0.1 M or 0. 1 N ceric sulfate until the red color is changed to pale blue. From the volume of 0.1 N ceric sulfate consumed, calculate the molarity/normality.

Hydrochloric acid (0.1 M or 0.1 N)

HCl   36.46

36.46 g in 1000 ml

Dilute 8.5 ml of hydrochloric acid with water to 1000 ml. Standardize the solution as follows.

Weigh accurately 0.1 g of anhydrous sodium carbonate (previously heated at about 250°C for 1 hour in an oven). Dissolve in 30 ml of water in a 250 ml conical flask. Add 0.1 ml of methyl red solution as indicator. Add hydrochloric acid slowly from a burette, with constant stirring until solution becomes faintly pink. Heat the solution to boiling,

$$Na_2CO_3 + 2HCl \rightarrow 2NaCl + H_2O + CO_2$$

Cool and continue the titration until the faint pink color is no longer affected by continued boiling. Calculate the molarity/normality of hydrochloric acid.

$$\text{Molarity / Normality} = \frac{\text{Weight of Na}_2\text{CO}_3\,(\text{g})}{0.053 \times V\,(\text{ml of acid used})}$$

Hydrochloric acid (0.5 M or 0.5 N) in methanol

HCl   36.46

18.23 g in 1000 ml

To a 1000 ml volumetric flask containing 40 ml of water slowly add 43 ml of hydrochloric acid. Cool, and add methanol to volume. Standardize the solution as directed under *hydrochloric acid, normal* (1 N), beginning with "Dissolve in 50 ml of water."

Iodine (0.05 M or 0.1 N)

I   126.90

12.69 g in 1000 ml

Dissolve about 14 g of iodine in a solution of 36 g of potassium iodide in 100 ml of water, add 3 drops of hydrochloric acid, dilute with water to 1000 ml, and standardize the solution as follows.

Transfer 25 ml of the iodine solution to a 250 ml flask, dilute with water to 100 ml, add 1 ml of 1 N hydrochloric acid, swirl gently to mix, and titrate with 0.1 M or 0.1 N sodium thiosulfate until the solution has a pale yellow color. Add 2 ml of starch mucilage indicator and continue titrating until the solution is colorless. Calculate the molarity/normality.

Preserve in amber-colored, glass-stoppered bottles.

Lead nitrate (0.1 M)

Pb(NO$_3$)$_2$ 331.21

33.12 g in 1000 ml

Xylenol orange triturate: Triturate 1 part of xylenol orange with 99 parts of potassium nitrate.

0.1 M lead nitrate: Dissolve 33 g of lead nitrate in 1000 ml of water. Standardize the solution as follows. To 20 ml of the lead nitrate solution add 300 ml of water. Add about 50 mg of xylenol orange triturate, and add methenamine until the solution becomes violet-pink. Titrate with 0.1 M edetate disodium to the yellow endpoint. Calculate the molarity.

Lithium methoxide (0.02 M or 0.02 N) in methanol

CH$_3$LiO   37.97

759.6 mg in 1000 ml

Dissolve 0.12 g of freshly cut lithium metal in 150 ml of methanol, cooling the flask during addition of the metal. When the reaction is complete, add 850 ml of methanol, and mix. Store the solution preferably in the reservoir of an automatic delivery buret suitably protected from carbon dioxide and moisture. Standardize the solution by titration against benzoic acid as described under sodium methoxide (0.01 M or 0.1 N) (in toluene), but use only 100 mg of benzoic acid. Each 2.442 mg of benzoic acid is equivalent to 1 ml of 0.02 M or 0.02 N lithium methoxide. [**Note:** Restandardize the solution frequently.]

> **Lithium methoxide (0.1 M or 0.1 N) in benzene**
>
> CH_3OLi 37.97
>
> 3.798 g in 1000 ml

Dissolve 0.6 g of freshly cut lithium metal in 150 ml of methanol, cooling the flask during addition of the metal. When reaction is complete, add 850 ml of benzene. If cloudiness or precipitation occurs, add sufficient methanol to clarify the solution. Store preferably in the reservoir of an automatic delivery buret suitably protected from carbon dioxide and moisture. Standardize the solution by titration against benzoic acid as described under sodium methoxide (0.1 M or 0.1 N) (in toluene). [**Note:** Restandardize the solution frequently.]

> **Oxalic acid (0.05 M or 0.1 N)**
>
> $H_2C_2O_2.2H_2O$ 126.07
>
> 6.303 g in 1000 ml

Dissolve 6.45 g of oxalic acid in water to make 1000 ml. Standardize by titration against freshly standardized 0.02 M or 0.1 N potassium permanganate as directed under potassium permanganate, (0.02 M or 0.0.1 N). Preserve in glass-stoppered bottles, protected from light.

> **Perchloric acid (0.1 M or 0.1 N) in glacial acetic acid**
>
> $HClO_4$ 100.46
>
> 10.05 g in 1000 ml

Mix 8.5 ml of perchloric acid with 500 ml of glacial acetic acid and 21 ml of acetic anhydride, cool, and add glacial acetic acid to make 1000 ml. Alternatively, the solution may be prepared as follows. Mix 11 ml of 60% perchloric acid with 500 ml of glacial acetic acid and 30 ml of acetic anhydride, cool, and add glacial acetic acid to make 1000 ml. Allow the prepared solution to stand for 1 day for the excess acetic anhydride to be combined., and determine the water content by Karl Fischer method. If the water content exceeds 0.5%, add more acetic anhydride. If the solution contains no titratable water, add sufficient water to obtain a content of between 0.02% and 0.5% of water. Allow the solution to stand for 1 day, and again titrate the water content. The solution so obtained contains between 0.02% and 0.5% of water, indicating freedom from acetic anhydride.

Standardize the solution as follows:

Weigh accurately about 700 mg of potassium biphthalate, previously crushed lightly and dried at 120°C for 2 hours, and dissolve it in 50 ml of glacial acetic acid in a 250 ml flask. Add 2 drops of crystal violet indicator and titrate with the perchloric acid solution until the violet color changes to blue-green. Deduct the volume of the perchloric acid consumed by 50 ml of the glacial acetic acid, and calculate the molarity/normality. Each 20.42 mg of potassium biphthalate is equivalent to 1 ml of 0.1 N perchloric acid.

> **Potassium bromate (0.01667 M or 0.01 N)**
>
> $KBrO_3$ 167.00
>
> 2.784 g in 1000 ml

Dissolve 2.784 g of potassium bromate in water to make 1000 ml, and standardize the solution as follows.

Transfer an accurately measured volume of about 40 ml of the solution to a glass-stoppered flask, add 3 g of potassium iodide, and follow with 3 ml of hydrochloric acid. Allow to stand for 5 minutes, then titrate the liberated iodine with 0.1 N sodium thiosulfate, adding 3 ml of starch mucilage indicator as the endpoint is approached. Correct for a blank run on the same quantities of the same reagents, and calculate the molarity/normality.

Potassium bromide–bromate (0.1 N)

Dissolve 2.78 g of potassium bromate ($KBrO_3$) and 12.0 g of potassium bromide (KBr) in water, and dilute with water to 1 000 ml. Standardize by the procedure set forth for potassium bromate (0 .1 N).

Potassium dichromate (0.06 M or 0.1 N)

$K_2Cr_2O_7$ 294.18

4.903 g in 1000 ml

Dissolve about 5 g of potassium dichromate in 1000 ml of water. Standardize the solution as follows.

Transfer 25.0 ml of this solution to a glass-stoppered, 500 ml flask, add 2 g of potassium iodide (free from iodate), dilute with 200 ml of water, add 5 ml of hydrochloric acid, allow to stand for 10 minutes in a dark place, and titrate the liberated iodine with 0.1 M or 0.1 N sodium thiosulfate, adding 3 ml of starch mucilage indicator as the endpoint is approached. Correct for a blank run on the same quantities of the same reagents, and calculate the molarity/normality.

Potassium ferricyanide (0.05 M)

$K_3Fe(CN)_6$ 329.24

16.46 g in 1000 ml

Dissolve about 17 g of potassium ferricyanide in water to make 1000 ml. Standardize the solution as follows.

Transfer 50 ml of this solution to a glass-stoppered, 500 ml flask, dilute with 50 ml of water, add 10 ml of potassium iodide and 10 ml of dilute hydrochloric acid, and allow to stand for 1 minute. Then, add 15 ml of zinc sulfate solution (1 in 10), and titrate the liberated iodine with 0.1 M or 0.1 N sodium thiosulphate, adding 3 ml of starch mucilage indicator as the endpoint is approached.

Protect from light, and restandardize before use.

Potassium hydroxide (1 M or 1 N)

KOH 56.11

56.11 g in 1000 ml

Dissolve 68 g of potassium hydroxide in about 950 ml of water. Add a freshly prepared saturated solution of barium hydroxide until no more precipitate forms. Shake the mixture thoroughly, and allow it to stand overnight in a stoppered bottle. Decant the clear liquid, or filter the solution in a tight, polyolefin bottle, and standardize by the procedure set forth for sodium hydroxide (1 M or 1 N).

> **Potassium hydroxide, methanolic (0.1 M or 0.1 N)**
> 5.612 g in 1000 ml

Dissolve about 6.8 g of potassium hydroxide in 4 ml of water, and add methanol to make 1000 ml. Allow the solution to stand in a tightly stoppered bottle for 24 hours. Then quickly decant the clear supernatant liquid into a suitable, tight container, and standardize the solution as follows.

Measure accurately about 25 ml of 0.1 M or 0.1 N hydrochloric acid. Dilute with 50 ml of water, add 2 drops of phenolphthalein and titrate with the methanolic potassium hydroxide solution until a permanent, pale pink color is produced. Calculate the normality. [**Note:** Store in tightly-stoppered bottles, protect from light.]

> **Potassium iodate (0.05 M)**
> KIO_3 214.00
> 10.70 g in 1000 ml

Dissolve 10.7 g of potassium iodate, previously dried at 110° to constant weight, in water to make 1000 ml.

> **Potassium permanganate (0.02 M or 0.1 N)**
> $KMnO_4$ 158.03
> 3.161 g in 1000 ml

Dissolve about 3.3 g of potassium permanganate in 1000 ml of water in a flask, and boil the solution for about 15 minutes. Insert the stopper in the flask, allow it to stand for at least 2 days, and filter through a fine-porosity, sintered-glass crucible. If necessary, the bottom of the sintered-glass crucible may be lined with a pledget of glass wool. Standardize the solution as follows.

Accurately weigh about 200 mg of sodium oxalate, previously dried at 110° to constant weight, and dissolve it in 250 ml of water. Add 7 ml of sulfuric acid, heat to about 70°, and then slowly add the permanganate solution from a buret, with constant stirring, until a pale pink color, which persists for 15 seconds, is produced. The temperature at the conclusion of the titration should be not less than 60°. Calculate the molarity/normality. Each 6.7 mg of sodium oxalate is equivalent to 1 ml of 0.02 M or 0.1 N potassium permanganate.

Since potassium permanganate is reduced on contact with organic substances such as rubber, the solution must be handled in apparatus entirely of glass or other suitably inert material. It should be frequently restandardized. Store in glass-stoppered, amber-colored bottles.

> **Silver nitrate (0.1 M or 0.1 N)**
> $AgNO_3$ 169.87
> 16.99 g in 1000 ml

Dissolve about 17.5 g of silver nitrate in 1000 ml of water, and standardize the solution as follows.

Transfer about 100 mg, accurately weighed, of reagent-grade sodium chloride, previously dried at 110°C for 2 hours, to a 150 ml beaker, dissolve in 5 ml of water, and add 5 ml of acetic acid, 50 ml of methanol, and about 0.5 ml of eosin indicator. Stir, preferably with a magnetic stirrer, and titrate with the silver nitrate solution. Calculate the molarity/normality.

> **Sodium arsenite (0.05 M)**
>
> NaAsO$_2$ 129.91
>
> 6.496 g in 1000 ml

Transfer 4.9455 g of arsenic trioxide, which has been pulverized and dried at 100° to constant weight, to a 1000 ml volumetric flask, dissolve it in 40 ml of 1 M or 1 N sodium hydroxide, and add 0.5 M or 1 N sulfuric acid or 1 M or 1 N hydrochloric acid until the solution is neutral or only slightly acid to litmus. Add 30 g of sodium bicarbonate, dilute with water to volume, and mix.

> **Sodium hydroxide (1 M or 1 N)**
>
> NaOH   40.00
>
> 40.00 g in 1000 ml

Accurately weigh about 5 g of potassium biphthalate, previously crushed lightly and dried at 120°C for 2 hours, and dissolve in 75 ml of carbon dioxide-free water. Add 2 drops of phenolphthalein indicator and titrate with the sodium hydroxide solution to the production of a permanent pink color. Each 204.2 mg of potassium biphthalate is equivalent to 1 ml of 1 M or 1 N sodium hydroxide.

[Notes: (i) Solutions of alkali hydroxides absorb carbon dioxide when exposed to air. They should be preserved in bottles having well-fitted, suitable stoppers, provided with a tube filled with a mixture of sodium hydroxide and lime (soda-lime tubes) so that air entering the container must pass through this tube, which will absorb the carbon dioxide. (ii) Prepare solutions of lower concentration (e.g. 0.1 N, 0.01 N) by quantitatively diluting accurately measured volumes of the 1 M or 1 N solution with sufficient carbon dioxide-free water to yield the desired concentration.] Restandardize the solution frequently.

> **Sodium hydroxide, alcoholic (0.1 M or 0.1 N)**
>
> NaOH   40.00

To 250 ml of alcohol, add 2 ml of a 50% (w/w) solution of sodium hydroxide.

Dissolve about 200 mg of benzoic acid, accurately weighed, in 10 ml of alcohol and 2 ml of water. Add 2 drops of phenolphthalein indicator and titrate with the alcoholic sodium hydroxide solution until a permanent pale pink color is produced. Calculate the molarity/normality as follows:

$$W/(122.12\ V)$$

in which W is the weight, in mg, of benzoic acid taken, V is the volume, in ml, of alcoholic sodium hydroxide consumed, and 122.12 is the molecular weight/equivalent weight of benzoic acid.

> **Sodium methoxide (0.1 M or 0.1 N) in toluene**
>
> CH$_3$ONa   54.02
>
> 5.402 g in 1000 ml

Cool in ice-water 150 ml of methanol contained in a 1000 ml volumetric flask, and add, in small portions, about 2.5 g of freshly cut sodium metal. When the metal has dissolved, add toluene to make 1000 ml, and mix. Store preferably in the reservoir of an automatic delivery buret suitably protected from carbon dioxide and moisture. Standardize the solution as follows.

Accurately weigh about 400 mg of primary standard benzoic acid, and dissolve in 80 ml of dimethylformamide in a flask. Add 3 drops of a 1 in 100 solution of thymol blue indicator in dimethylformamide, and titrate with the sodium methoxide to a blue endpoint. Correct for the volume of the sodium methoxide solution consumed by 80 ml of the dimethylformamide, and calculate the molarity/normality. Each 12.21 mg of benzoic acid is equivalent to 1 ml of 0.1 M or 0.1 N sodium methoxide.

[**Notes:** (i) To eliminate any turbidity that may form following dilution with toluene, add methanol (25 to 30 ml usually suffices) until the solution is clear. (ii) Restandardize the solution frequently.]

Sodium nitrite (0.1 M or 0.1 N)

$NaNO_2$ 69.00

6.900 g in 1000 ml

Dissolve 7.5 g of sodium nitrite in water to make 1000 ml, and standardize the solution as follows.

Accurately weigh about 500 mg of sulfanilamide RS, previously dried at 105° for 3 hours, and transfer to a suitable beaker. Add 20 ml of hydrochloric acid and 50 ml of water, stir until dissolved, and cool to 15°. Maintaining the temperature at about 15°, titrate slowly with the sodium nitrite solution, placing the buret tip below the surface of the solution to preclude air oxidation of the sodium nitrite, and stir the solution gently with a magnetic stirrer, but avoid pulling a vortex of air beneath the surface. Use the indicator specified in the individual monograph, or, if a potentiometric procedure is specified, determine the endpoint electrometrically, using platinum-calomel or platinum-platinum electrodes. When the titration is within 1 ml of the endpoint, add the titrant in 0.1 ml portions, and allow 1 minute between additions. Calculate the molarity. Each 17.22 mg of sulfanilamide is equivalent to 1 ml of 0.1000 M sodium nitrite.

Sodium tetraphenylboron (0.02 M)

$NaB(C_6H_5)_4$ 342.22

6.845 g in 1000 ml

Dissolve an amount of sodium tetraphenylboron, equivalent to 6.845 g of $NaB(C_6H_5)_4$, in water to make 1000 ml, and standardize the solution as follows.

Pipet two 75 ml portions of the solution into separate beakers, and to each add 1 ml of acetic acid and 25 ml of water. To each beaker add, slowly and with constant stirring, 25 ml of potassium biphthalate solution (1 in 20), and allow to stand for 2 hours. Filter one of the mixtures through a filtering crucible, and wash the precipitate with cold water. Transfer the precipitate to a container, add 50 ml of water, shake intermittently for 30 minutes, filter, and use the filtrate as the saturated potassium tetraphenylborate solution in the following standardization procedure. Filter the second mixture through a tared filtering crucible, and wash the precipitate with three 5 ml portions of saturated potassium tetraphenylborate solution. Dry the precipitate at 105°C for 1 hour. Each g of potassium tetraphenylborate is equivalent to 955.1 mg of sodium tetraphenylboron. From the weight of sodium tetraphenylboron obtained, calculate the molarity of the sodium tetraphenylboron solution.

[**Note:** Prepare this solution fresh.)

Sodium thiosulfate (0.1 M or 0.1 N)

$Na_2S_2O_3 \cdot 5H_2O$ 248.19

24.82 g in 1000 ml

Dissolve about 25 g of sodium thiosulfate and 200 mg of sodium carbonate in 1000 ml of recently boiled and cooled water. Standardize the solution as follows.

Accurately weigh about 210 mg of primary standard potassium di chromate, previously pulverized and dried at 120°C for 4 hours, and dissolve in 100 ml of water in a glass-stoppered, 500 ml flask. Swirl to dissolve the solid, remove the stopper, and quickly add 3 g of potassium iodide, 2 g of sodium bicarbonate, and 5 ml of hydrochloric acid. Insert the stopper gently in the flask, swirl to mix, and allow to stand in the dark for exactly 10 minutes. Rinse the stopper and the inner walls of the flask with water, and titrate the liberated iodine with the sodium thiosulfate solution until the solution is yellowish green in color. Add 3 ml of starch mucilage indicator and continue the titration until the blue color is discharged. Perform a blank determination . Calculate the molarity/normality.

Sulfuric acid (0.05 M or 0.1 N)

H_2SO_4 98.08

49.04 g in 1000 ml

Add slowly, with stirring, 3.0 ml of sulfuric acid to about 1000 ml of water, allow to cool to 25°, and determine the molarity/normality by titration against sodium carbonate as described under hydrochloric acid.

Tetrabutylammonium hydroxide (0.1 M or 0.1 N)

$(C_4H_9)_4NOH$ 259.47

25.95 g in 1000 ml

Dissolve 40 g of tetra-*n*-butylammonium iodide in 90 ml of anhydrous methanol in a glass-stoppered flask. Place in an ice bath, add 20 g of powdered silver oxide, insert the stopper in the flask, and agitate vigorously for 60 minutes. Centrifuge a few ml, and test the supernatant liquid for iodide. If the test is positive, add an additional 2 g of silver oxide, and continue to allow to stand for 30 minutes with intermittent agitation. When all of the iodide has reacted, filter through a fine-porosity, sintered-glass funnel. Rinse the flask and the funnel with three 50 ml portions of anhydrous toluene, adding the rinsings to the filtrate. Dilute with a mixture of three volumes of anhydrous toluene and 1 volume of anhydrous methanol to 1000 ml, and flush the solution for 10 minutes with dry, carbon dioxide-free nitrogen. [**Note:** If necessary to obtain a clear solution, further small quantities of anhydrous methanol may be added.] Store in a reservoir protected from carbon dioxide and moisture, and discard after 60 days. Alternatively, the solution may be prepared by diluting a suitable volume of commercially available tetrabutylammonium hydroxide solution in methanol with a mixture of 4 volumes of anhydrous toluene and 1 volume of anhydrous methanol. [**Note:** If necessary to obtain a clear solution, further small quantities of methanol may be added.]

Standardize the solution on the day of use as follows. Dissolve about 400 mg of primary standard benzoic acid, accurately weighed, in 80 ml of dimethylformamide, add 3 drops of a 1 in 100 solution of thymol blue indicator in dimethylformamide, and titrate to a blue endpoint with the tetrabutyl-ammonium hydroxide solution, delivering the titrant from a buret equipped with a carbon dioxide absorption trap. Perform a blank determination, and make any necessary correction. Each ml of 0.1 M or 0.1 N tetrabutylammonium hydroxide is equivalent to 12.21 mg of benzoic acid.

> **Zinc sulfate (0.05 M)**
>
> $ZnSO_4 \cdot 7H_2O$ 287.56
>
> 14.4 g in 1000 ml

Dissolve 14.4 g of zinc sulfate in water to make 1 litre. Standardize the solution as follows.

Measure accurately about 10 ml of 0.05 M edetate disodium into a 250 ml conical flask, and add, in the order given, 10 ml of acetic acid-ammonium acetate buffer, 50 ml of alcohol, and 2 ml of dithizone Titrate with the zinc sulfate solution to a clear, rose-pink color. Calculate the molarity

APPENDIX II (A)

CONCENTRATED REAGENTS, MOLARITY AND NORMALITY

Concentrated reagents	Density	Molarity (M)	Normality (N)	Volume (ml) required to make 1000 ml solution	
				1 M	1 N
Acetic acid 99.5%	1.05	17.4	17.4	57.5	57.5
Ammonia 35%	0.880	18.1	18.1	55.3	55.3
Ammonia 25%	0.910	13.4	13.4	74.6	74.6
Hydrochloric acid 36%	1.18	11.65	11.65	85.8	85.8
Hydrochloric acid 32%	1.16	10.2	10.2	98.0	98.0
Hydrofluoric acid 40%	1.13	22.6	22.6	44.2	44.2
Nitric acid 70%	1.42	15.8	15.8	63.3	63.3
Perchloric acid 60%	1.54	9.2	9.2	108.7	108.7
Perchloric acid 70%	1.67	11.6	11.6	86.2	86.2
Orthophosphoric acid 85%	1.7	15.2	45.6	65.8	21.9
Sodium hydroxide 47%	1.5	17.6	17.6	56.7	56.7
Sulfuric acid 98%	1.84	18.4	36.8	54.3	27.2

APPENDIX II (B)

REAGENTS AND THEIR MOLARITY AND NORMALITY

Reagents	Molecular weight	Equivalent weight	'g' required to make 1000 ml	
			1 M	1 N
As_2O_3	197.14	49.26	197.14	49.26
$CaCO_3$	100	50	100	50
Ceric ammonium nitrate, $Ce(NO_3)_4.2NH_4NO_3$	548.22	548.22	548.22	548.22
Ferrous ammonium sulfate, $Fe(NH_4)_2(SO_4)_2.6H_2O$	392.13	392.13	392.13	392.13
Ferric ammonium sulfate, $Fe(NH_4)(SO_4)_2.12H_2O$	482.19	482.19	482.19	482.19
Iodine, I_2	253.80	126.90	253.80	126.90
Oxalic acid, $(COOH)_2.2H_2O$	126	63	126	63
Potassium iodate, KIO_3	214	35.66	214	35.66
Potassium bromate, $KBrO_3$	167.0	27.83	167.0	27.83
Potassium permanganate, $KMnO_4$	158.04	31.60*	158.04	31.60*
Potassium hydroxide, KOH	56	56	56	56
Potassium dichromate, $K_2Cr_2O_7$	294.18	49.03	294.18	49.03
Sodium chloride, NaCl	58.5	58.5	58.5	58.5
Sodium carbonate. Na_2CO_3	106	53	106	53
Sodium hydroxide, NaOH	40	40	40	40
Sodium bicarbonate, $NaHCO_3$	84	84	84	84
Sodium nitrite, $NaNO_2$	69	69	69	69
Sodium thiosulfate, $Na_2S_2O_3.2H_2O$	248.19	248.19	248.19	248.19
Silver nitrate, $AgNO_3$	169.18	169.18	169.18	169.18

* In acidic medium

APPENDIX III

pH INDICATORS

pH indicators are usually weak acids or weak bases that change their color depending on their dissociation (protonation) state. Sometimes both forms are colored, sometimes only one.

pH indicators—colors and color change pH range

Indicator name	pH/Color	pH/Color	Indicator name	pH/Color	pH/Color
Brilliant green	0.0 Yellow	2.6 Green	Litmus	5.0 Red	8.0 Blue
Eosin yellowish	0.0 Yellow	3.0 Green fluoresc.	Bromocresol purple	5.2 Yellow	6.8 Purple
Erythrosine B	0.0 Yellow	3.6 Red	Bromophenol red	5.2 Orange/yellow	6.8 Purple
Methyl green	0.1 Yellow	2.3 Blue	4-Nitrophenol	5.4 Colorless	7.5 Yellow
Methyl violet	0.1 Yellow	2.7 Violet	Bromoxylenol blue	5.7 Yellow	7.5 Blue
Cresol red	0.2 Red	1.8 Yellow	Bromothymol blue	6.0 Yellow	7.6 Blue
Crystal violet	0.8 Yellow	2.6 Blue/violet	Phenol red	6.4 Yellow	8.2 Red/violet
m-Cresol purple	1.2 Red	2.8 Yellow	3-Nitrophenol	6.6 Colorless	8.6 Yellow/orange
Thymol blue	1.2 Red	2.8 Yellow	Neutral red	6.8 Blue/red	8.0 Orange/yellow
p-Xylenol blue	1.2 Red	2.8 Yellow	Creosol red	7.0 Orange	8.8 Purple
Eosin, bluish	1.4 Colorless	2.4 Pink fluoresc.	1-Naphtholphthalein	7.1 Brownish	8.3 Blue/green
Quinaldine red	1.4 Colorless	3.2 Pink	m-Cresol purple	7.4 Yellow	9.0 Purple
Bromochlorophenol blue	3.0 Yellow	4.6 Blue/violet	Thymol blue	8.0 Yellow	9.6 Blue
Bromophenol blue	3.0 Yellow	4.6 Blue/violet	p-Xylenol blue	8.0 Yellow	9.6 Blue
Congo red	3.0 Blue	5.2 Yellow/orange	Phenolphthalein	8.2 Colorless	9.8 Red/violet
Methyl orange	3.1 Red	4.4 Yellow/orange	Thymolphthalein	9.3 Colorless	10.5 Blue
Bromocresol green	3.8 Yellow	5.4 Blue	Alizarin yellow GG	10.0 Bright yellow	12.1 Brown/yellow
Alizarin sulphonic acid	4.3 Yellow	6.3 Violet	Indigo carmine	11.5 Blue	13.0 Yellow
Methyl red	4.4 Red	6.2 Yellow/orange	Titan yellow	12.0 Yellow	13.0 Red
Chlorophenol red	4.8 Yellow	6.4 Purple			

APPENDIX IV

SIGNIFICANT FIGURES

Experimental measurements

Whenever experimental measurements are made, there is always the possibility for errors in the reported value. These errors can arise because of one or more of the following.

1. Some type of limitation related to the nature of the measuring device;
2. Some error that can be attributed to the individual; and
3. Some type of approximation included in the measurement. Therefore, when numerical data are reported or interpreted, care must be exercised to produce the reliable data.

Consider the following examples of obtaining the mass of some object as an illustration of the statements made in the preceding paragraph. Suppose that the mass of an object is determined by using a triple-beam balance. The scales of many triple-beam balances are calibrated so that the mass can be read from the balance to the nearest 0 .1 g. Thus, the mass of the object would be reported as 15.3 g.

The mass 15.3 g can be interpreted as follows: The last number represents the least accurate digit in the determination . The mass of the object is definitely 15 g, but there is some uncertainty about the fractional portion. However, the fractional portion of the mass is approximately 0.3 g. A common practice of expressing this uncertainty is to assume or report that the correct value is within some range. The range is determined by taking one- half of the smallest value that can be read from the measuring device and showing that the correct value could deviate by this amount on either side of the reported value. Thus, since the smallest value which can be read from the triple-beam balance is 0.1 g, any weighing will be uncertain within the range of± 1/2 (0 .1) or ± 0.05 g. This means that for the weighing of the object that is reported at 15 .3 g, the correct mass would be in the range of 15.25 g to 15 .35 g.

If the mass of the same object was determined by using an analytical balance instead of the triple-beam balance, then the mass might be reported to be 15.3276 g. This piece of datum indicates that the uncertainty lies in the 0.0001 g place or that the mass of the object lies in the range of 15.32755 g and 15.32765 g.

Significant figures

The term "significant figures" is used to designate the number of digits contained in some datum which reflect the precision of the datum. The number of "significant figures" is determined by adding the number of digits contained in the datum. For example, when the mass of an object is reported as 15.3 g, there are three significant figures contained in the datum 15.3 g. When the mass is reported as 15.3276 g, there are six significant figures.

When zeros are part of numerical data, the determination of whether the zero is a significant digit or not will depend on the way the number is written and/or the location of the zeroes. Note the examples in Table 1.

Frequently, very large numbers or very small numbers are best written in terms of scientific notation. In this manner, the correct number of significant figures can be expressed most easily

Table 1

Number	Significant figures	Explanation
706	3	—
760	2	Since the decimal is not shown, the last figure with meaning is the 6 and the zero shows the magnitude
7.6×10^2	2	This is a better way to write 760
760	3	The zero is now significant because the location of the decimal has been specified!
7.60×10^2	3	Zeroes at the end of fractional numbers are significant
0.000206	3	The first 3 zeroes only locate the decimal, the middle zero is part of the number and therefore significant
2.06×10^{-4}	3	A better way to write 0.000206
$2.060 \ 10^{-4}$	4	The final zero is significant in that it shows the last digit that can be measured

Rounding-off

Often a number with a large number of significant figures should be expressed using a smaller number of significant figures. Consequently, a procedure called "rounding-off" is employed to reduce the number of significant figures. This procedure involves the dropping of all digits which are not considered to be significant and if required by convention, to add one to the last significant digits.

The following is an outline of the procedure to follow.

1. Determine the desired number of significant digits.
2. Examine the first digit after the last significant figure.
3. If this digit is less than 5, all the numbers after the last significant figure are dropped
4. If the digit described in 2 is greater than 5, all the numbers after the last significant figure are dropped, and the last significant figure is increased by one.
5. If the digit described in 2 is equal to 5, then the last significant figure is increased by 1 if it is an odd number, or left unchanged if it is an even number. Zero is considered to be an even number. (Note: If additional digits follow the 5, the last significant figure is increased by 1.)

The process is illustrated by the examples in Table 2.

Table 2

Number	Desired number of significant figures	Rounded-off number
3.732473	5	3.7325
1.483	3	1.48
8765	3	8760
8775	3	8780
11.637	4	11.64
1.6753	3	1.68

Arithmetic operations and significant figures

A means of recognizing the limitation of some measured quantity is by using the number of significant figures. Thus, the mass of an object as determined to be 15.3 g on a triple-beam balance has only three significant figures and the uncertainty is easily recognized.

Frequently, measured quantities are used to determine other quantities by calculation. Consequently the data are subjected to a variety or sequence of arithmetic operations. A calculated result must only contain the number of digits equal to the least accurate datum used.

Addition and subtraction

When a group of measured quantities are added or subtracted, the result must be expressed to reflect the least certain value. For example: Suppose that the total mass of a flask, a liquid placed into the flask, and a covering for the flask is to be determined. The values obtained by using different balances are:

Flask	257 g
Liquid	1.023 g
Cover	2.360 g
Total	260.383 g

In the above, the datum that has the least certainty (least precision) is the mass of the flask, i.e. it is only expressed to the nearest gram. Therefore, the final result can only be expressed to the nearest whole gram, i.e., total mass = 260 g.

Multiplication and division

The result of any series of multiplications and divisions can only be expressed using the number of significant figures equal to that number with the least significant figures. For example: evaluate the following.

$$\frac{(2.7 \times 10^{-3}) \times 377}{8.75} = 116.33 \times 10^{-3}$$

When the data are examined, the following can be determined: 2.7×10^{-3} has only two significant figures and the other numbers have three significant figures. Therefore, the result can only be expressed to two significant figures: 0.12.

Index

251